This book is so comforting to read! A wonderful exhortation to embrace our bodies' limits and receive God's gifts in rest.

—Justin Whitmel Earley, founder and CEO, Avodah Legal; author, *The Body Teaches the Soul*, *Habits of the Household*, and others

Sometimes I've wondered why sleep is part of God's design for the world we live in. I tend toward activity. I like to do things. Brett McCracken helps me see compelling reasons for valuing and embracing sleep and rest. Through Scripture and science, this book is both informative and inspiring. It's another McCracken book filled with practical wisdom.

—Mark Vroegop, president, The Gospel Coalition; author of multiple books, including *Dark Clouds, Deep Mercy: Discovering the Grace of Lament*

McCracken has penned what is perhaps the most complete, illustrative, and inspiring exploration of sleep to date in the Christian world. Weaving together biblical and theological wisdom—with a knack for pastoral sensitivity and care—he shows us the glorious joys of getting to worship the creator of human rest and sleep. Indeed, God's people worship the Lord of the Sabbath. Until we learn this, we won't rightly enter the life of work God has called us to.

—A. J. Swoboda (PhD, University of Birmingham), associate professor of Bible and theology, Bushnell University; pastor, Faith Center, Eugene, Oregon; author of many books, including *Subversive Sabbath*

This book is a gracious gift for weary souls. With clarity, humility, and theological care, McCracken helps us see sleep in a fresh way, not simply as a necessary pause from productivity but as a beautiful invitation to the freedom of limits and the comfort of trust. Brett lovingly reminds us that "life is not a debt we must work to pay off. It's a gift to receive." This is a much needed book for our overworked world.

—Jay Y. Kim, pastor; author, *Analog Church*

I bet you never thought about what sleep can teach you, both about yourself and about God. But the truth is, sleep is a gift from our Creator and a spiritual discipline for us. In this accessible book, McCracken takes us on this journey, offering wise reflections while always taking us back to our God, who is the Lord of our sleep.

—Kelly M. Kapic, author, *You're Only Human*; professor of theology, Covenant College

It is no small matter that when God revealed his top ten commands for humans to enjoy a covenantal relationship with their Creator, he included rest. As with so many other areas in which science is slowly catching up with age-old biblical insights, we find the blessing of sleep. With a masterful blend of biblical exposition and the latest science, along with pastoral wisdom, art, pop culture, and practical liturgies for the reader to apply, McCracken has done a great service to a weary church. His page-turning book will put us to sleep, but only in the best and most blessed way we all need.

—Dr. Thaddeus Williams, professor of theology, Biola University; author, *Revering God*, *Don't Follow Your Heart*, and *Confronting Injustice without Compromising Truth*

Humans appreciate the benefits of sleep only once it becomes elusive. When sleep flees, the psalms about crying out to God in the night become relevant, and the essential role that sleep plays in creatures' lives comes into focus. McCracken provides great insight on this role from a theological, physiological, and doxological perspective. He not only demonstrates that the wise value sleep, he shows what our need for sleep tells us about our Maker, the only wise God.

—Betsy Childs Howard, editor, The Gospel Coalition; author, *God Gives Sleep*

"Now I lay me down to sleep, I pray the Lord my soul to keep." Maybe it has been a long time since you've heard that bedtime prayer, but this book will remind you what a meaningful request it is, and what a gracious gift sleep is from our Creator. As usual, McCracken's ability to synthesize theology, biblical studies, intellectual history, philosophy, and the latest in sleep science is uncanny. But we, his readers, are the beneficiaries. Read this book and sleep tight.

—Matthew J. Hall, provost, Biola University

Unlike your fitness tracker, this book won't guilt-trip you about how much sleep you are getting. But it will remind you how something so simple—something we do every day—can habituate us to a God of grace who bids our strivings cease each time we lay down our heads. In a frenetic age, we need now more than ever to renew our minds and bodies with the formative rhythms of rest McCracken holds out to us in these pages. Perhaps then we can offer more genuinely to a weary and watching world the hope we say we believe in: that because Christ's work is finished, we can rest in the midst of ours.

—Whitney K. Pipkin, journalist, author, and editor

I am learning that the crux of sanctification is a willingness to lay down our arms. Everyone wants healthy habits, and most seek to love their neighbors, but only those captivated by Christ's love can understand that ultimately we are called to rest. This process has proven so difficult—or maybe it's just that I'm so obtuse—that I need to be reminded of it daily. In this book, McCracken provides a compelling reason to remember that the life we dream about is possible if only we trust that God provides even while we sleep.

—Jairo Namnún, teaching pastor, Cornerstone Church of Santo Domingo

Across his many clear-eyed and generous books, McCracken promotes health—what a healthy church looks like, how to have healthy disagreements, what a healthy relationship to technology is—so I suppose it is no surprise he has turned his attention to the subject of sleep, which, we are increasingly finding, is the root of nearly all health and healing.

And yet it is a surprise. Who knew the Scriptures offer so much guidance and good sense on a topic so quotidian? This book is, ironically, a wake-up call to be intentional about our sleep and sabbath practices, which leave us at our creaturely best, we who are called—commanded even—if sometimes to be watchful, also to rest.

—Dr. Mischa Willett, author of several poetry books;
director, Whitworth Writers Workshop

THE WISDOM OF SLEEP

How Rest Reveals God's Truth and Revives Weary Souls

BRETT MCCRACKEN

ZONDERVAN REFLECTIVE

ZONDERVAN REFLECTIVE
The Wisdom of Sleep

Published by Zondervan, 3950 Sparks Drive SE, Suite 101, Grand Rapids, MI 49546, USA. Zondervan is a registered trademark of The Zondervan Corporation, L.L.C., a wholly owned subsidiary of HarperCollins Christian Publishing, Inc.

Requests for information should be addressed to customercare@harpercollins.com.

Zondervan titles may be purchased in bulk for educational, business, fundraising, or sales promotional use. For information, please email SpecialMarkets@Zondervan.com.

ISBN 978-0-310-17572-5 (audio)

Library of Congress Cataloging-in-Publication Data

Names: McCracken, Brett, 1982– author
Title: The wisdom of sleep : how rest reveals God's truth and revives weary souls / Brett McCracken.
Description: Grand Rapids, MI, USA : Zondervan Reflective, [2026] | Includes bibliographical references. | Audience term: Christians
Identifiers: LCCN 2026016653 (print) | LCCN 2026016654 (ebook) | ISBN 9780310175711 paperback | ISBN 9780310175728 ebook
Subjects: LCSH: Sleep—Religious aspects—Christianity | Rest—Religious aspects—Christianity | Spiritual life—Christianity
Classification: LCC BV4598.13 .M33 2026 (print) | LCC BV4598.13 (ebook)
LC record available at https://lccn.loc.gov/2026016653
LC ebook record available at https://lccn.loc.gov/2026016654

Published in association with the literary agency of Wolgemuth & Wilson.

HarperCollins Publishers, Macken House, 39/40 Mayor Street Upper, Dublin 1, D01 C9W8, Ireland (https://www.harpercollins.com)

Cover design: Darren Welch
Cover image: ©CSA-Printstock / Getty Images
Interior design: Sara Guild

Printed in the United States of America

26 27 28 29 30 LBC 5 4 3 2 1

To Witt,

as he wakes to the world God made

Psalm 121:3–4

CONTENTS

INTRODUCTION

Sleep Talking: The Gospel Is Rest

The hour of rest approaches,
The toils of day are past,
And o'er our tired bodies
Sleep's gentle charm is cast.
—Prudentius, "Hymn Before Sleep"

Come to me, all you who are weary and
burdened, and I will give you rest.
—Matthew 11:28

Sometimes I wonder if heaven will feel a bit like an afternoon nap.

I have oddly specific memories of naps from decades ago. I remember the Sunday afternoon naps of my adolescence, when following our postchurch pot roast I retired to the basement and drifted away on our 1980s-style sectional sofa. I remember falling asleep on the couch watching the Masters. (Naps to the background noise of golf are the best.) I remember summers at a family camp in Lake Geneva, Wisconsin, when I would escape the afternoon humidity to nap in my parents' cabin, soothed by a rotating floor fan.

Why do I remember these mundane naps so specifically? And why, when they come to mind, do I feel a *Sehnsucht* tingling in my heart—that haunting feeling C. S. Lewis describes in *The Weight of Glory* as an "inconsolable longing" for a "far-off country . . . for something that has never actually appeared in our experience"?[1]

Maybe it's because naps are signposts of something far greater that we've not yet fully experienced. Maybe it's because even the most relaxing vacation, replenishing Sabbath, and restorative night's sleep are only teasers for the perfect rest we're wired to desire. Maybe there's more to sleep and rest than we think. Maybe in his mysterious sovereignty, God designed these things to be a sacred portal of sorts, a connective tissue between heaven and earth, between death and resurrection, between the God of rest and the restless souls who can't help but be magnetically tugged toward him.

In a world driven by constant productivity, a nap can feel like the rarest of gifts and the most unnecessary of splurges—a bracketed-off break from the steady stream of stresses, notifications, and tasks that populate our lives. Especially for those who struggle to sleep and feel tired almost constantly, the purity of a satisfying snooze can feel heavenly.

It's the backyard hammock on the perfect spring day; the couch in a cabin as autumn rain and leaves fall outside; that stolen time every parent feels when the kids are all elsewhere, the house is (momentarily) quiet and clean, and nothing demands our attention except the stillness of slumber for a small stretch of time.

A nap can feel like grace. An unearned and unexpected gift.

It can feel like the temporal equivalent of what the Celts called thin places, where the veil between heaven and earth feels strangely sheer.

ETERNITY IN A DAY, OR A DREAM

Some of life's greatest mysteries concern our conflicted relationship with time. If time—life lived chronologically, at a fixed pace—is perfectly normal, why do we feel pain at its passage? Why are there so many mysterious, inexplicable anomalies with time (for example, *déjà vu*)? Why do some days feel like weeks and some weeks like days? Why do certain moments feel holy and set apart (what the Greeks called *kairos*) from the normal experience of time (*chronos*)? And why does time do such weird things in our sleep and dreams?

This last dynamic, like my surprising remembrance of specific naps decades ago, is a clue that there's something deeper at play in the phenomenon of sleep.

You know the sensation. You fall asleep and wake up, and it feels like only seconds have passed. But you've slept for seven hours. Or you dream so expansively that when you wake, it feels like you've just had a decade's worth of experiences. You're so disoriented by the entire life you've just lived in your sleep that it takes a minute to reorient.

What's up with this? Could it be that the mysterious realm of sleep is a place where God shakes us out of time and pulls us toward eternity, giving us daily glimpses in our time-bound lives of the time-unbound future we can one day have with him?

Perhaps God is doing a similar thing in his design for a day of rest he made holy (Gen. 2:3) and called his people to keep holy (Ex. 20:8; Deut. 5:12). In Ezekiel 20 he instructs his people to "keep my Sabbaths holy, *that they may be a sign* between us. Then you will know that I am the LORD your God" (Ezek. 20:20, emphasis added). God seems to want his people to constantly remember eternity—to remember him. So as in sleep, so in Sabbath: He provides what Abraham Heschel calls "a window in eternity that opens into time."[2]

A sign. A portal. A foretaste. A gift.

COME, ALL WHO ARE WEARY

In this book, I will explore how God communicates with us through our experiences of sleep, rest, and Sabbath. But it's not just impersonal communication *about* himself. It's relational communication that invites us *into* himself. It's communication toward the end of communion with him.

Jesus says, "Come to me" for rest (Matt. 11:28). He doesn't say "I will give you rest" as if it were a gift he orders on Amazon and has shipped to your home. No, rest is more than a present. It's found in his presence. Jesus' goal in rest is not just to give you a break. It's to give you himself. The more we are in Christ, the more we are at rest.

This invitation—for weary souls to accept his invitation to enter into rest in him—captures the heart of what the gospel is and does.

The gospel is a free gift. Our salvation is received, not achieved. In an exhausted world burdened by sin, temptation, ceaseless toil, and ever-present trouble, God invites us to rest in him. Having purchased our peace and eternal rest through the death and resurrection of his Son, Jesus Christ, God invites us into green pastures by still waters. If you struggle with sleep, waking in the night with racing thoughts, as I sometimes do, it's not because you've fallen on God's bad side. Remember: God is for you; he wants to bring you to a place that knows no insomnia, anxiety, fear, or scarcity, but only an overflowing cup (Psalm 23).

The gospel is rest.

We desperately need this reminder. In his song "The Gospel Is Rest," Christian artist Elias Dummer fittingly repeats the phrase, "Oh, how I need it." He speaks for all of us. We've always needed the gospel of rest. But oh, how we need it in today's excruciatingly burdened, hyperexhausted, increasingly anxious world.

Though it's not true for everyone, humans today generally enjoy more comfortable, less interrupted sleep than our forebears, when climate-controlled dwellings weren't a thing and sleeping conditions were often dangerously cold. At the same time, we're probably the least rested generation in human history. So much in modern life, both within us and around us, leaves us deeply tired on a soul level, if not always on a physical level.

We're exhausted by the onslaught of information, push notifications, task-management tools, obsession with productivity, and the ubiquitous buzz of algorithmic consumerism. We're exhausted by foolishness on social media and the Ecclesiastes-style vanity of life in a scrolling world. We're exhausted by internal expectations to achieve and external expectations to produce. We're exhausted by our flesh's frailty—the Romans 7 tendency to keep doing what's wrong while struggling to do what's right.

We're exhausted by the hustle-and-grind mindset that proposes constant work as the norm and all else as laziness. We're exhausted by individualism and its lonely burdens: the widespread expectation that each of us needs to find our true self and express it in some memorable, distinct way. We're exhausted by the self and its constant, often-warped need to be liked, loved, known, seen, respected, affirmed, understood. We're exhausted by how social media fosters an obsessive pressure to capture, record, post, and perform. We're exhausted by the litany of sorrows, questions, comparisons, and outrages that confronts us daily when we open our phones. We're exhausted by the tension of desiring the "far-off country," yet only being able to glimpse it faintly, weary as we are in a world of toil, thorns, thistles.

Life has always been hard under the sun. Weariness is as old as life East of Eden, when our fallen ancestors were first exiled from the perfect rest of God. But in a technological age bent on anesthetizing our ache for Eden with elixirs of amusement and stimulants of "optimized time," life under the sun feels especially hot. Oh, how we need shade!

Thankfully, God is our shade (Ps. 121:5), and he built relief into the rhythm of creation. Even though he "will neither slumber nor sleep" (v. 4) himself, he gives us the gift of sleep. Life is brutal under the sun. But every day the sun sets. Every day the moon rises. And by God's grace, what does night bring but a chance to die and rise again via replenishing sleep, a reset that can feel like a cleansing breeze across the bay from Paradise lost.

UNIVERSALITY OF SLEEP

Sleep is something we all do. This is not a topic exclusive to the leisure class or those who can afford a (typically very expensive) wellness lifestyle. It's a universal part of human experience, a fundamental rhythm in our creational identity. Sleep is not just a pleasant thing we get to do, nor is it a necessary evil we frequently struggle to do. Neither is sleep merely fuel for the two-thirds of our lives when we're awake and active.

Sleep has immense restorative utility and is unparalleled in its mysterious power to replenish and heal the body. Summarizing the latest research on sleep's many benefits, neuroscientist Matthew Walker argues that sleep "is the single most effective thing we can do to reset our brain and body health each day," noting that the question for scientists is no longer what sleep is "good for" but rather "whether there are any biological functions that do *not* benefit by a good night's sleep."[3]

We'll look at the science of sleep later in this book, but for now, here's a question to ponder: What does it mean that God created us such that the single most effective thing we can do for our biological flourishing is not something we can work at or earn but rather the passive activity of stillness and deathlike sleep? All the work we put in at the gym, all the meticulous calorie counting, all the kale smoothies and charcoal cleanses and essential oils—these surely bring *some* health benefit. But they pale in comparison with the simply received grace of a good night's sleep.

In the "death" of sleep, when our strivings literally cease, we find the greatest gains of life and strength. Is this not another way in which sleep speaks gospel truth?

NECESSITY OF THE UNNECESSARY

The God we worship is a God of overflowing extravagance and limitless abundance. Sleep and rest are unnecessary gifts. God could have created us to be always-on, always-working machines. Instead he created us to have substantial periods of rest. What superfluous grace! And when we receive these good gifts and happily pause to rest during the week and sleep during the night (even if our sleep is often far from perfect), we show our gratitude and bear witness to a reality beyond brute efficiency, productivity, and results. We bear witness to a God of abundance and the spacious peace that is possible for all who trust in him.

That's what this book is about: how our rest points to his glory. It's about how something like sleep can be part of what the Westminster Shorter Catechism calls "the chief end of man": "to glorify God, and to enjoy him forever."

The book is structured in two parts, inspired by Calvin's notion that wisdom "consists almost entirely of two parts: the knowledge of God and of ourselves."[4] Part 1 ponders what sleep and rest reveal about us: our limitations and our possibilities, according to God's design. Part 2 moves into reflections on what sleep and rest reveal about God, the wise and beneficent designer of these gifts. At the end of each chapter is a "Pause" prompt: a brief action or practical step to take in response. I include these in the hope that the ideas explored in the book aren't just interesting to you but life-altering in tangible ways. I also include questions for you to ponder—whether by yourself or as part of a group discussion. Since sleep is something everyone does—and yet is full of challenges and mysteries—I suspect this book could be especially stimulating to read and discuss with others.

As you read, I hope you're provoked to love and worship God more, grateful for the gospel of rest and the teasers of perfect peace he gives us here and now. I hope you're inspired to enter more fully into joyful, restful communion with God, such that the witness of your life piques the curiosity of unbelievers looking for a real respite in the hectic chaos of life. For all who are weary and heavy laden, I pray this book draws you further into the rest offered by the Lord of the Sabbath.

Part 1

WHAT SLEEP AND REST REVEAL ABOUT US

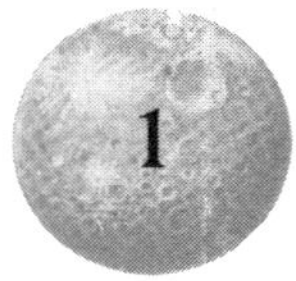

1

SLEEP'S DEEP

We're Wired to Seek Meaning

Sleep, the main course in life's feast, and the most nourishing.
—William Shakespeare, *Macbeth*

I lie down and sleep;
I wake again, because the Lord sustains me.
—Psalm 3:5

Why do we sleep? What is the meaning of this rather odd thing that we daily do, from before we are born until our dying day? Humans have pondered these questions for millennia. It's almost like we're wired to wonder about the why behind the prominent features of our design.

Sleep occupies a huge portion of every human's existence. And as far as scientists have discovered, all animals sleep, rest, or exhibit sleeplike behavior. Yet as much as science has uncovered a lot of what sleep is and what it does, consensus on the central why of this universal phenomenon remains frustratingly elusive.

WHAT SLEEP AND REST REVEAL ABOUT US

A strictly materialist worldview interprets biological phenomena in terms of evolutionary advantage. For secular scientists, the meaning of sleep is not poetic or philosophical; it can be understood only in utilitarian terms—what a function does for creatures such that it would have evolved so universally and persisted so stubbornly across time.

Certainly science has discovered much that sleep does for creatures. The litany of health benefits is quite impressive. Every year, researchers discover new, compelling evidence of the ways sleep restores bodies and brains. We'll look at those discoveries throughout this book. But the central why and "evolutionary necessity" of sleep remains a curiously unanswered question. Here's how some leading sleep scientists express the conundrum:

> We have known the functions of the three other basic drives in life—to eat, to drink, and to reproduce—for [many] years now. Yet the fourth main biological drive, common across the animal kingdom—the drive to sleep—has continued to elude science for millennia.[1]

> The reasons why we sleep remain frustratingly unresolved. Many explanations have been proposed, but no one overarching hypothesis has emerged to explain why this major aspect of our behavior exists.[2]

> Everybody knows that sleep is important, yet the function of sleep seems like the mythological phoenix . . . nobody has yet identified a core function of sleep.[3]

If anything, sleep seems foolish in a survival-of-the-fittest world, a liability more than an asset. If natural selection logically favors a creature's ability to find food, mate and reproduce, and protect offspring, those are all things that can't be done during sleep. Sleep is a highly exposed state, leaving creatures vulnerable to predators or other dangers that would seem to be a high evolutionary cost relative to whatever benefits sleep might provide.

These significant liabilities complicate the scientific question of why sleep is so ubiquitous across time and space. Sleep is clearly not a mistake of nature, but what is its primary benefit for our survival that makes it worth all the costs? Some leading evolutionary theories for the core function of sleep include (1) cellular restoration, (2) energy conservation, and (3) the consolidation of memory and learning. But there are compelling counterarguments for each of these.[4]

Even if scientific consensus on sleep's necessity remains elusive, there is unanimous agreement that sleep is helpful. Some scientists describe sleep as "useful without being essential."[5] But from a strictly materialist perspective, "useful without being essential" feels pretty shaky, especially for something as universal and biologically consequential as sleep. Sleep is not anomalous in nature. It's a prominent feature, a deep structure supporting life across the animal kingdom. This is why researchers are still in hot pursuit of the holy-grail answer of sleep's central why.[6]

American philosopher Sara Protasi recently pondered a thought experiment: What if there were a "rest pill" we could take that "could make us skip sleep altogether and get all the benefits of a full night of sleep. Should we take it?"[7] If we see ourselves as machines defined merely by our productivity and functional outputs, we'd probably say yes. But Protasi argues that sleep's value goes beyond its utility (which is real!). There's a *meaning* to sleep that is deeply tied to being human: "Sleeping's underlying biological need is not a weakness to be remedied, or a limitation to be overcome, but a fact of our nature that gives rise to valuable interpersonal and aesthetic activities and is also valuable in itself. If we never slept, our lives would be deprived of an important source of meaning and goodness."

Machines can't appreciate the meaning and goodness of their operation; robots can't ponder the gracious elegance of their design. But humans can. And we do. We have a built-in curiosity about the higher logic and beautiful generosity of our design. We can't help but wonder, What if sleep exists for reasons that defy utilitarian logic? What if the helpful and useful aspects of sleep are better explained by creational grace than evolutionary science? Could it be that the reason evolutionary science struggles to fully explain sleep is because there are layers and mysteries to sleep that can't be fully explained by evolutionary theory?

TWO BOOKS, ONE AUTHOR

For centuries, Christians have spoken of Scripture and nature/creation as "two books" containing God's "special revelation" (Scripture) and "general revelation" (creation). Since they are authored by the same creator, we shouldn't be surprised to find common themes, motifs, and parallels between the two books. Indeed, God's communication in Scripture often uses the material realities of creation (the second book) to help readers understand spiritual truths. Consider Jesus' parables, in which he frequently uses nature imagery to illustrate the kingdom. God's world helps reinforce the truths of God's Word. Once you start looking at creation with that in mind, you see connections everywhere.

This is why something like sleep—which might seem so mundane and familiar as to be unworthy of deeper consideration—begs to be examined through a theological lens. The book of nature tells us a lot about the glorious benefits of sleep. But for the meaning and ultimate why of sleep's existence, we need the book of

Scripture. We need to be able to move beyond natural selection and also talk about supernatural intention. In God's infinite wisdom, he saw fit to build some form of rest or sleep into the design of all living creatures. He found it "very good" to create humans to spend one-third of their lives sleeping.

Isn't that striking? God made us so that one-third of our lives is spent doing nothing but lying flat, eyes closed, unproductive, and passively receiving the gift of replenishing repose. He designed us so that daily we assume a physical state that bears unmistakable resemblance to death, only to "resurrect" hours later feeling miraculously energized and enlivened. In our sleep-wake cycle we enact nothing less than the gospel arc itself: not just life after death but life from death.

This raises the question why. There is so much to unpack here, not only from the fascinating science of sleep but also from the ways in which sleep shows up in the Bible and the theological threads that connect it to the broader theme of Sabbath rest. For God did not just design us to sleep one-third of our lives. He also desires that we rest on a Sabbath day, one-seventh of each week. In both his specially revealed commands and generally revealed creation, rest is a theme God chooses to emphasize. We should take note.

This is not to say we should sleep our lives away or live only for the weekend. We are still awake more than we are asleep, by God's design. We still work six out of the seven days a week, by God's design. There are good endeavors and important tasks for us to do. We shouldn't spend every moment merely waiting for (or practicing for) the eternal Sabbath to come. Sleep is a gift to relish, but sleeping too much can lead to the sin of sloth.

Still, we should not be so frantically consumed by the tasks, trials, and triumphs of life in time that we lose the perspective of eternity. Perhaps God designed the biology of sleep and the rhythm of Sabbath as daily and weekly ways to keep the everlasting rest of heaven perpetually in view. They are reminders of heaven not only in their goodness but also in their "not yet" imperfection. Sleep can be a struggle, after all. Deep rest is often elusive.

Sleep and rest are also God-designed, built-in teachers of humility. It's human nature, after all, to become convinced of our own importance. We're inclined to want to justify our existence by accomplishing great things. But sleep and rest are God's whispers to us that doing isn't everything. Sometimes we are to be still and know he is God (Ps. 46:10). To be at peace in his safety (Ps. 4:8). To be with him as a branch abides in the vine (John 15:4). To be.

Life is not a debt we must work to pay off. It's a gift to receive.

SLEEP'S WISDOM, ACCORDING TO SCRIPTURE *AND* SCIENCE

Much can be illuminated when we combine the insights of general revelation with the truths of special revelation. Contrary to the tired narrative that faith and science are in conflict, God's Word and God's world are a powerful interpretative combo for making sense of things like sleep (among other mysteries of creation). That's the approach we'll take throughout this book, which is a devotional and practical work of "creational theology."[8]

We'll draw insights on sleep and rest from both the book of Scripture and the book of creation, which cannot contradict one another since they're written by the same infallible author. If scientific and Christian claims about reality seem in conflict, we must conclude that one side is simply reading reality wrong. There is only one reality: God's. And it cannot be in conflict with itself. The study of God's world (science) and the study of God's Word (theology) should be mutually enriching disciplines because they're studying the work of the same creator.

I've found this to be true as I've read both scientific and theological perspectives on sleep. Both offer valuable and complementary insights, even as their fundamental suppositions about reality might differ. As I hear sleep scientists marvel at the impressive, interconnected ways sleep contributes to holistic health, I get the sense that they want to call it miraculous and give thanks to *someone* for such a mind-blowing, beneficial gift. Yet to whom or to what can they give thanks? Christian faith gives us a worthy object. Christianity provides a paradigm of transcendence that makes satisfying sense of immanent wonders. When science reveals new complexities at the cellular level or new mysteries at the intergalactic level, it only reinforces our awe at the Creator's genius; it only reinvigorates our worship and desire to know him more.

Humans are wired to seek meaning beyond the materialist horizon. We've never been satisfied simply to accumulate empirical observations and facts about the world—however fascinating and jaw dropping they are. We want to know what it all means. What it's for.

Evolutionary atheism offers scientific theories for why humans like music, why humans cry and laugh, and why we find sunsets and waterfalls beautiful. But most people find these survival-advantage explanations cold and unsatisfying. We intuitively know utilitarian explanations for these things can't be the whole story. We resonate when Bon Iver sings, "There are things behind things behind things."[9] We sense earthly reality is charged with meaning that goes deeper than mere survival and contains a logic that goes beyond mere function. There are layers of meaning to excavate beneath almost every surface appearance. With its telescopes and microscopes, science helps us look closer. But faith can help us go deeper. Science excels at discovering the marvelous whatness of things. Faith helps us with the whyness.

For Christian theists (which includes many scientists!), the meaning of earthly things goes beyond earthly reality. We look at the natural world not as a cold, dead place that meaninglessly stumbled into mind-boggling intricacy over untold eons but as a painstakingly crafted cosmos that reflects and glorifies a creator. As Rémi Brague puts it, "Natural things have a meaning. They are not only just there, at our disposal, but can convey a message and become our teachers."[10]

To be sure, nature *is* at our disposal and *does* offer useful benefits for *this* world. But nature doesn't exist for its own sake. Every creation has a purpose and meaning beyond itself. Van Gogh's *Starry Night* doesn't exist for its own sake as merely canvas with pigment. It exists to lead us to ponder the real starry nights above us every day. It points beyond itself. And the real starry night, likewise, doesn't exist for its own sake as merely a collection of lonely, innumerable giant balls of hot gas trillions of miles from one another. They too point beyond themselves, as King David knew (Ps. 8:3–5). They point to the Creator.

It's what Paul is getting at in Romans 1: "For since the creation of the world God's invisible qualities—his eternal power and divine nature—have been clearly seen, being understood from what has been made, so that people are without excuse" (Rom. 1:20).

R. C. Sproul calls this "mediate revelation," because it is revelation that comes to us via the medium of nature, making visible "the invisible power and deity of God himself."[11] John Calvin similarly describes "the elegant structure of the world," which serves as "a kind of mirror, in which we may behold God, though otherwise invisible." Echoing Paul in Romans 1, Calvin says, "On each of his works his glory is engraved in characters so bright, so distinct, and so illustrious, that none, however dull and illiterate, can plead ignorance as their excuse."[12] His glory is engraved on *each* of his works. Not just the flashy ones (galaxies, grand canyons, northern lights) but also the mundane ones.

Like sleep.

So let's look closer and consider how a natural phenomenon like sleep is more than the sum of its utilitarian biological parts but is also "an earthly picture of a spiritual reality"[13] with meaning beyond itself. Sleep, rest, yawns, dreaming—they are all brushstrokes on the Creator's canvas, artistic choices that may seem peculiar, but are doubtless intentional.

These are artistic choices begging for us to ask, What kind of artist would incorporate these motifs of sleep and rest so prominently in his work? And how do these motifs serve his overarching creative goal? Put another way, what do sleep and rest reveal about who God is? And what do they reveal about God's purposes for us?

These questions will animate the rest of this book.

Pause and Ponder

Pause

Think about your history with sleep. What memories come to mind of childhood bedrooms, college dormrooms, or other places you've slept? Are there particular dreams or nightmares you remember? Spend two minutes writing down words you associate with sleep. They could be nouns (for example, specific places), adjectives describing your felt experience of sleep, or anything. Don't overthink it; just write whatever comes to mind in two minutes or less. Then look at your list and reflect on your associations with sleep coming into this book.

Ponder

1. Where else have you seen examples of how "God's world helps reinforce the truths of God's Word"? Is there some phenomenon in nature that has enriched your understanding of a theological truth or an attribute of God?
2. If the book of Scripture and the book of creation "cannot contradict one another since they're written by the same infallible author," why do you think faith and contemporary science are perpetually butting heads?
3. As you begin this book, how would you characterize your relationship with sleep? Do you sleep well, or struggle to sleep? What are your biggest pain points with sleep?
4. Have you ever given thought to the meaning of sleep and rest as brushstrokes on the Creator's canvas?

2

NODDING OFF

We're Limited

I've always loathed the necessity of sleep. Like death,
it puts even the most powerful men on their backs.
—Frank Underwood, in Netflix's *House of Cards*

But God chose the foolish things of the world
to shame the wise; God chose the weak things
of the world to shame the strong.
—1 Corinthians 1:27

I love planning elaborate trip itineraries. I spend hours researching landmarks, museums, hikes, hotels, restaurants, shops, coffee shops, Google Maps walking routes, and more in the hope of crafting a perfectly curated experience that maximizes every minute of our time. But I've learned over the years—especially since becoming a dad with now four young kids—that maximization cannot be my utmost value. A maximized itinerary usually backfires.

WHAT SLEEP AND REST REVEAL ABOUT US

A few years ago, we went on a three-week trip driving all over the Colorado Rocky Mountains with kids who were four, three, and one. (Crazy? Maybe.) It was mostly a lot of fun. But there were definitely some not-fun moments that typically resulted from my ambitious, grueling pace.

On one day in particular, as we were transferring from the Boulder area to Breckenridge, my desire to do everything almost did us in. I had us drive one hour from Boulder to do a hike to Mitchell Lake, which ended up being a longer and harder hike than we anticipated. (Two adults carrying three kids on backs, you know.) Exhausted and hot, from there we still had to drive two hours to Silverthorne, where I had ordered a birthday cake from a bakery. (It was my middle son's third birthday that day, on top of everything else!) My plan was for us to pick up the cake, get some food at a grocery store, and then drive the final thirty minutes to our Breckenridge Airbnb, where we hoped to arrive before dinnertime and have a nice little birthday celebration.

But since we hadn't really had lunch, the kids were starving and we had to add an unplanned late-afternoon stop for food. Then the grocery shopping took longer and was more stressful than expected. By the time we finally arrived at our Airbnb, it was nearly dark, my blood pressure was off the charts, and everyone was miserable. I had pushed us too hard—favoring optimization over enjoyment—and we all knew it. I had basically ruined my son's birthday. I felt terrible.

From that experience and others like it, I've learned that having young kids on family trips imposes necessary limitations: shorter outings, easier hikes, a looser schedule, and above all, blocks of time for naps. Overtired kids can make even the best vacation go haywire in a hurry. Do we get to see and do everything we want to see and do within these limitations? No. But I've come to love vacation naps and rest times. It's good to have downtime. Breathing room. Even in beautiful places where there's no end to what you could be exploring, it's good to make space to be still.

ANOMALY OF REST IN AN ALWAYS-ON WORLD

Technology is gradually rendering rest and downtime anomalous.

It started with the invention of the lightbulb. Nighttime illumination made it possible for commerce, transportation, and all manner of activities to persist 24-7. But the internet took the always-on world to the next level. The hyperconnected online world hums with activity at all hours: ecommerce, social media, content creation and consumption, streaming media. TV channels used to cease broadcasting at the end of the day, usually before midnight local time. Now every channel has constant programming. News is broadcast 24-7, despite the fact that there's simply not enough newsworthy information to fill a never-ending broadcast.

These technological changes have also blurred the boundaries of work and home. With email, Slack, Asana, and text messages knowing no temporal limitations, more and more of us are never really off the clock. No rest until the inbox is tamed! (The inbox is never tamed.) Can't sleep at 1:00 a.m.? Grab the device on your nightstand and start scrolling, your bleary-eyed face aglow in blue-white LED light in a room meant for sleeping.

Today, established rhythms of rest and sleep can feel like antiquated luxuries. We can still choose to prioritize them. But it's no longer the cultural expectation.

The inconvenient truth in an always-on world, however, is that sooner or later we do have to turn off. All-nighters might occasionally work when you're twenty-one, but even then, they're ill-advised. Attempting to subsist on the bare minimum of sleep may work for a season, but it will catch up with you in your long-term health. (More on that in the next chapter.) When you fly across time zones and your circadian rhythm is out of whack, you can try to manage it with melatonin or other hacks. But jet lag will always affect you. We are meant to rest and sleep in regular intervals. When we don't, things go awry.

IN ACHIEVEMENT CULTURE, REST IS WEAKNESS

Our low view of rest and sleep also stems from a growing cultural pressure to optimize, maximize, and hustle to gain competitive advantage. Rest less, strive more. It's the "sleep when I'm dead" mentality. Rest is for losers.

In *The Burnout Society*, Byung-Chul Han observes that we live in an "achievement society" rather than a "disciplinary society." People are now "entrepreneurs of themselves," driven by an open-ended "imperative to achieve." The watchword is *can*. The world is your oyster. The sky's the limit. It's a world where "prohibitions, commandments, and the law are replaced by projects, initiatives, and motivation." The problem, however, is that this "nothing is impossible" pressure to achieve causes exhaustion, depression, and burnout. "Depression is the sickness of a society that suffers from excessive positivity," Han argues.[1] One becomes depressed, Alain Ehrenberg adds, "because he must tolerate the illusion that everything is possible for him."[2]

An overinflated sense of what we can achieve through productivity—a limitlessness to our can-do ambition—leads to weariness.

Inevitably we are confronted with the brute fact of our finitude. There are some things we can't do.

This is a blow to our pride. Thomas à Kempis once said, "A proud and avaricious man never rests."[3] Trusting in our own capacities leads us to a restless pursuit of more, better, bigger. Yet the need for rest is a relentless ghost haunting even the most high-capacity people. Sleep is "the balancing weight that levels the shepherd with the king, and the simple with the wise," declares Sancho Panza in *Don Quixote*.[4]

Sleep and rest know no hierarchies. They are egalitarian impositions. Elon Musk needs sleep as much as Taylor Swift does, as much as bus drivers in Bangladesh do. Even mighty men like Samson are vulnerable in sleep, as Judges 16 makes clear. Even Jesus needed rest and sleep (Matt. 8:24; Mark 4:38; Luke 8:23). It was part of his full humanity.

Still, the temptation toward godlike limitlessness is real.

PUSHING OUR LIMITS

You don't have to look far to see contemporary loathing for limits. From Netflix's Chris Hemsworth series, *Limitless*, to the "Unlimited" mantra of *Wicked*'s "Defying Gravity," to the sexual revolution's demands for bodily autonomy, to the expectation for "unlimited calls and texts!" cell phone plans, it's everywhere.

Limitlessness is an intoxicating sales pitch. It has been since Eden.

We see the desire to transgress boundaries in our cultural fixation on setting athletic records and conquering new frontiers of space and time. We see it in "playing God" technologies that create and design babies through technologies like IVF and gene editing.

We see it in political efforts to deregulate commerce, protect free speech from any limitation, and ensure the individual's rights to decide who they marry, what gender they want to be, and whether they want to end an unwanted pregnancy.

Digital technology makes the "limitless" illusion more real. Online, we can pretty much go anywhere, say anything, be anyone, buy anything, find any information we desire. The smartphone, AI, and the internet are humanity's closest-yet approximations of godlike omnipotence, omniscience, and omnipresence. The more we live in virtual spaces, the more the limitations of our bodies recede. We can be scrolling in virtual space at night and the next thing we know, it's past midnight and our bodies' tiredness finally shakes us out of our LED-light trance. In the disembodied digital age, it's not surprising that transgenderism feels plausible. In online life, our bodies have no bearing on our identities or actions. So we start to apply this online logic offline too, declaring that who we really are has no necessary connection to the biological limitations connected to male or female bodies.[5]

In *The Extinction of Experience*, Christine Rosen argues that the digital world has turned us into disembodied users rather than finite, embodied individuals: "Our current technologies . . . persuade us that we can opt out of bodily limitations in ways that even the invention of the telegraph, telephone, automobile, and jet airplane did not. . . . We have created technologies that so effectively extend our senses that we have started mistrusting the signals our physical bodies give us."[6]

There's a neo-Gnosticism at play here. Christians, who believe God knew what he was doing when he created us with limited bodies, should be the first to reject digital life's illusion of disembodied limitlessness. Yet Christians can sometimes be just as deceived as anyone by secular tenets such as unbridled freedom, bodily autonomy, and a "no sleep until I'm dead" obsession with achievement.

Well-meaning Christians can associate sleeplessness with godliness, reading into proverbs about sluggards (for example, Prov. 6:6–11; 10:4–5; 19:15; 26:14) a wholesale devaluing of sleep and rest. Examples from church history can also make it seem like sleeping as little as possible is a holy calling: monks waking up at dawn for prayer (Lauds), heroes like Hudson Taylor or George Whitefield rising before day to read and pray,[7] and countless Christian leaders modeling a preference for "redeeming the time" over getting seven hours of nightly sleep.

Habitual devaluing of sleep is unbecoming for Christians. We are not machines that simply need to be plugged in for a few hours each day to optimize the rest of our time. Rest is not merely utilitarian. God created it for a reason.

LIMITS OF YOUR CONTROL

Modernity's impulse is control. Technology helps bring more and more of the world's variables and challenges—disease, sickness, weather, geographical distance, securing food and water—under our domain. But total controllability is an illusion.

Some things in life stubbornly defy attempts at mastery—weather, for example. I wish I could snap my fingers and make it rain. I can't. In Southern California, where I live, we can go seven or eight months without rain, heightening the risk for cataclysmic wildfires. In a drought I often pray for soaking rainstorms, knowing only this "act of God" will ultimately prevent or extinguish massive fires. But this is not something we can force to our will. It's a grace God gives, or doesn't.

Our need for rest and sleep is another one of these things. We can do our darndest to bring this realm under technological control: sleeping pills to fall asleep, coffee and energy drinks to stay awake, biometric-optimized sleep schedules, and more. But ultimately the body's needs, rhythms, and wiring overrule our wishes for convenience.

In *The Uncontrollability of the World*, Hartmut Rosa points to the moment of falling asleep as emblematic of his theory of resonance, which is the magic of the world that happens serendipitously and eludes our control: "We cannot bring [sleep] about simply by willing it. The more we want it, the less we get it, at least sometimes." It reminds me of something C. S. Lewis once said in a letter: "About sleep: do you find that the great secret (if one can do it) is not to *care* whether you sleep? Sleep is a jade who scorns her suitors but woos her scorners."[8]

The frustratingly uncontrollable onset of sleep, Rosa argues, contrasts with modernity's "incessant desire to make the world engineerable, predictable, available, accessible, disposable . . . in all its aspects." Rosa argues that resonance is inherently uncontrollable. No amount of hacks or interventions can determine its occurrence or its length. "Just as with falling asleep, the harder we try to make it happen, the less we succeed."[9]

Rosa's idea of resonance portrays uncontrollability not as a loss or a deficiency but as an opportunity. A gift. Sleep and rest are resonant because they come and go unpredictably and defy our attempts to fit them into some sort of maximizer's schedule. An unplanned, twenty-minute nap on the couch can be one of your most beautiful sleeps of the year. A planned-for-months vacation at a five-star resort might, unfortunately, contain some of your most restless nights ever. We can do some things to set our rest up for success: avoiding alcohol and caffeine before bed, going to bed at the same time each night, reading a physical book in bed instead of scrolling. But sometimes we can't do enough.

We are limited beings. That's a good thing.

SLEEP REMINDS US: LIMITS ARE A GIFT

In contrast to our culture's "Unlimited!" anthem, the truth is we *are* limited. We aren't the Creator (Job 38:4). We're creatures. We must live within rules, laws, and limits we didn't make. Far from godlike, we are dust quickly returned to dust, our days a fleeting shadow (Ps. 144:4). "Everyone is but a breath, even those who seem secure" (Ps. 39:5).

Our need for sleep reminds us. Even in moments when we really want to be awake, in spite of all the will we can muster, we can't stay awake. This is the central conceit that makes the Nightmare on Elm Street movies terrifying. The stalked teenagers in this franchise know that if they fall asleep, they'll probably become victims to Freddy Krueger's dreamworld killing spree. Yet sleep invariably comes for them in spite of their best efforts to stay awake. Tiredness always wins.

"Sleep is a spiritual discipline that daily reminds us of our lack of control," Kelly Kapic says. "It requires us to see our finitude as a good part of God's design for us."[10] Perhaps no biblical scene shows this as memorably as the moment in Gethsemane when Jesus brings Peter, James, and John with him and tells them to keep watch while he goes to pray (Mark 14:32–42). Even in this climactic moment of Jesus' mission, they can't stay awake. Their flesh is weak. They've been through a heavy night. They no doubt desire to stay awake for Jesus in his hour of greatest need. But sleep wins.

John Piper says God sends us to bed each night like patients who are ill with a sickness: "The sickness is a chronic tendency to think we are in control and that our work is indispensable. To cure us of this disease God turns us into helpless sacks of sand once a day. How humiliating to the self-made corporate executive that he has to give up all control and become as limp as a suckling infant every day."[11]

We can lament this reality as a weakness. Or we can see it as part of God's wisdom, for our good. God's wisdom, after all, sometimes looks like foolishness to the world. Christ crucified epitomizes this. Yet "the foolishness of God is wiser than human wisdom," Paul famously wrote, "and the weakness of God is stronger than human strength" (1 Cor. 1:25).

Our world sees power, strength, success, and achievement very differently than God does. Where the world calls us to conquer and "crush it!" on our own merits, God defines true power as Christ being "crushed for our iniquities" (Isa. 53:5), achieving our salvation for us, because of Christ's merits. Where the world operates on the Darwinian logic of survival of the fittest, Jesus calls his followers to turn the other cheek (Matt. 5:39) and take up their crosses daily (Luke 9:23). Where the world declares sleep a necessary annoyance at best, Scripture says it's something God gives to his beloved (Ps. 127:2).

Embrace the gift. Be humbled by your limits. Make peace with the uncontrollability of the world.

Pause and Ponder

Pause

Pinpoint one or two specific areas of your life where you struggle to give up control or accept limits. Talk with someone—a spouse, a friend, a pastor—about this and brainstorm ways you can embrace limits or loosen your control in these areas.

Ponder

1. How do you balance the good impulse to work hard and make the most of your time, with the bad expressions of optimization mentioned in this chapter? What are the warning lights that can indicate your life is geared a bit too much in the machine/user mindset rather than the limited-human mindset?
2. Where does the desire for controllability show up in your life?
3. Do you think sleep and rest are examples of the "weak things of the world" that shame the strong (1 Cor. 1:27)? In what specific ways do these things keep our pride and tempation toward godlike power in check?

3

DEAD ASLEEP

We're Mortal

Sleep serves as a daily *memento mori*, a reminder of our death.
—Tish Harrison Warren, *Prayer in the Night*

For dust you are
and to dust you will return.
—Genesis 3:19

Dead asleep." "Dead to the world." These euphemisms speak to the message sleep shouts: You're mortal. You will die.

Though waking up in the morning is a pleasant picture of resurrection, nightly slumber is a fearsome image of death. We assume a position that looks eerily like a corpse: lying flat, still, eyes closed, in an altered consciousness, somewhere else between the world our senses perceive and a realm that invades our dreams.

Sometimes sleep is too close to death for our comfort. I remember when our kids were infants, sleeping in bedside bassinets. They often looked so deep in sleep that we had to put our ears close to their faces or examine their little bodies to make sure we heard breathing or saw flinches of movement. Sleeping looks so much like death that people who die in their sleep are often discovered only in the morning. This is one reason nighttime was feared for much of human history. The space between life and death is thinnest in the darkest part of night.

Why did God create sleep to be so deathlike? He could have created a human rest posture that looked different: sitting up, eyes open, still. He could have made us like fish, with unihemispheric sleep: half our brain sleeping while the other half is awake, theoretically allowing us to be semiactive all the time. But he didn't. Instead, his design for our sleep is decidedly death-mimicking. And he's an intentional designer.

I think God wants us to keep our mortality in constant view. Sleep is a glorious gift for our rest, yes, but it's also a gift for our remembrance. We are mortal; our deaths are inescapable. Our numbered days like ephemeral dreams. Our "little life," Shakespeare famously wrote, "is rounded with a sleep."[1] Keeping this fact center stage is good for our wisdom (Psalm 90). *Memento mori.*

SLEEP, THE BROTHER OF DEATH

Humans have long recognized the close connection between sleep and death. In Greek mythology, the gods of sleep (Hypnos) and death (Thanatos) are twin brothers, sons of the goddess of night (Nyx). The brotherly association of sleep and death continued in early Christianity. Athenagoras, a second-century Athenian philosopher who converted to Christianity, postulated that sleep was like "the brother of death" not because the two shared the same mythological ancestry "but because those who are dead and those who sleep are subject to similar states, as regards at least the stillness and the absence of all sense of the present or the past, or rather of existence itself and their own life."[2] Early Christian theologian Tertullian called sleep the "mirror of death." And Scripture often uses *sleep* and *death* interchangeably (for example, John 11:11; Acts 7:60; 13:36; 1 Cor. 11:30). The closeness of sleep and death is undeniable in human and biblical history.

You might be wondering, though, if God created sleep in part to remind us of our mortality, what does it mean that sleep existed before the fall, before death as a consequence for sin became a thing? Was Adam's deep sleep in Genesis 2:21 a one-off sleep event, or was nightly sleep a regular thing for him and Eve before the fall? We do know night existed from the beginning (Gen. 1:5), as did rhythms of rest (Gen. 2:2). So sleep and circadian rhythms likely existed as a part of God's design for a good creation, even before sleep's mirror-of-death quality had a reference point in human death. Maybe for Adam and Eve, sleep's deathlike quality was an unknown signifier until the fall, when it suddenly became an unmistakable foreshadowing of their mortality.

In God's infinite creative wisdom, sleep can be a multipurposed phenomenon: simultaneously a wonderfully gracious gift and an ominous reminder of death. He created it, after all, with full knowledge of the reality of human mortality to come. As it exists for us now, it carries a multitude of meanings: a blessing, a mercy, and a relief; yet also a chastening, a humbling, and a warning.

A SMALL TASTE OF BIG SLEEP

Raymond Chandler famously associated sleep with death in his 1939 crime novel, *The Big Sleep*. On one hand this slang for death is an attempt, in an increasingly secular world, to soften its blow. Death will just be like going to sleep peacefully, but . . . forever.

However, the implications of this actually infuse our nightly sleep with *more* terror, reminding us that every sleep foreshadows the big sleep to come.

In a 2008 episode of *This American Life*, "Fear of Sleep," host Ira Glass ponders his own fear of sleep and unpacks reasons why others are terrified of bedtime, this "small taste of the big sleep."[3] Early in the program, Glass describes his fear: "As early as I remember, I was afraid to go to sleep. . . . I would lie awake at night, scared to fall asleep, because sleep seemed no different than death. You know. You were gone, not moving, not talking, not thinking, not aware—not aware. What could be more frightening?"

Later in the program Glass hears from others with similar fears. Here's what anonymous "Man 2" has to say: "It's not irrational fear. It's like you understand that you're mortal. Your life is going to be over at some point. You're fighting, like, the worst enemy in the world as you lie there in bed, rolling around in your sheet covers, in your blankets. And you're rolling around there, trying to fight death. And there's no way you can win."

This is the dread of sleep. We want to fight death, but we know we can't win. There's a deep vulnerability to it, a sense of being incapacitated, claustrophobic, as in a coffin with no escape. There's a frightening loneliness to it. When we go to sleep, it's our journey to take; no one else can take it for us. Each sleeper is an island. Sleep and death are solitary frights. As seventeenth-century English Puritan William Bates put it, "There is a natural love of society in man, and death removes from all. The grave is a frightful solitude. . . . Every one among the dead is confined to his sealed, obscure cell, and is alone an entertainment for the worms."[4]

Maybe this is one reason couples sleep in the same bed, and in many cultures and times in history entire families co-sleep together. Sleeping communally is a coping mechanism for the isolating terror of night, both practically (the safety of body heat in dangerously cold sleeping conditions) and existentially. Sleep researchers have also shown that the security we feel co-sleeping next to loved ones triggers the release of oxytocin, which helps us fall asleep faster and have longer, better quality sleep. Sleeping close to someone we love not only protects us but restores us as we sleep; it is an act of both intimacy and solidarity. Whatever comes in the night—however scary its foreshadowing of death—we'll face it together.

HOW CONTEMPORARY CULTURE COPES WITH DEATH

Community helps us face the reality of mortality in the same way it helps us cope with the terror of night. A 2025 Netflix documentary, *Don't Die*, illustrates this powerfully. The film follows tech millionaire Bryan Johnson, whose Project Blueprint seeks to "neutralize aging" through an intense regimen of biometric-data monitoring, hyperprescribed fitness routines, various electromagnetic therapies, gene manipulation, plasma infusions, and dozens of daily pills and supplements. Having retired from his career as a successful entrepreneur, abandoning the Mormon faith of his childhood and becoming estranged from his large family, Johnson now spends his time living in a solitary California mansion merely trying to extend his life (with the help of an expensive team of nutritionists and antiaging experts). His existence revolves around reversing his age and attempting to conquer the body's corruptibility.

This is a sad and futile quest. But what's fascinating about Johnson's story arc in *Don't Die* is how he comes to recognize how meaningless it is to prolong life if you live alone, without meaningful relationships. As the film goes on, Johnson seeks out connection with his college-age son and his father, as well as a growing online community he meets up with for organized hikes, runs, or Don't Die summits. In the documentary's final moments, we see groups of strangers all over the world wearing Don't Die T-shirts as they gather for antiaging microevents. The images strike me as illustrative of a secular culture coping with a deep fear of death and loneliness by finding solidarity in the attempt to overcome it.

Don't Die is part of a growing movement called transhumanism, a sci-fi philosophy that believes advanced technologies will one day defeat death and make human immortality possible. Even if most normal people don't go as far as transhumanist fantasies, your average person in the modern West *is* afraid of death and is trying to conquer it. Growing cottage industries of health and wellness, optimization, productivity, and bucket-list pleasure maximization are expressions of it.

It's this scarcity mentality driven by the fear of death that leads people to devalue rest and sleep. Adrian Reynolds believes contemporary culture's "low view of sleep—as something which just interrupts the real business of the day—may be reflective of a low view of death: you've got to pack as much in before you're finished."[5]

In their 2024 article "The Coddling of the American Funeral," Megan Starr and Noah Senthil suggest various other ways contemporary culture copes with fear of death:

> We've exchanged the mourning of death at funerals for the "celebration of life"; we've separated graveyards from church property and relegated them to memorial parks, hidden from view; and we've overwhelmingly chosen cremation (61.9 percent) rather than burial (33.2 percent), so we don't have to see dead bodies. Perhaps there's a cultural illusion that if we don't think about it, don't talk about it, and don't see it, it won't happen to us or our children. But it will. We're going to die.[6]

You see signs of contemporary culture's anxiety about death on the bestseller lists.

Peter Attia's *Outlive: The Science and Art of Longevity* is one prominent example. Yuval Harari's *Homo Deus: A Brief History of Tomorrow* is another. In an article at the onset of the 2020 COVID-19 pandemic—a time when modern Western culture was confronted with realities of human frailty in deeply uncomfortable ways—Harari defiantly insists that deadly diseases are merely "technical problems" that have "technical solutions." He laments that, for most of history, "the best human minds were busy giving meaning to death, not trying to defeat it." But after the scientific revolution, we now realize that "death isn't a divine decree—it is merely a technical problem."[7]

Other atheist thinkers deal with mortality not by overcoming it through science but by leaning in to its inevitability and seizing the day. This is the perspective of Swedish philosopher Martin Hägglund in his 2019 book, *This Life: Secular Faith and Spiritual Freedom*.[8] Hägglund recognizes the finitude of life but rejects any notion of life after death. But this finitude—"the sense of the ultimate fragility of everything we care about"—is for him precisely what gives life meaning. It is "the condition for anything to be at stake." This is at the heart of what he calls secular faith, as opposed to religious faith. Religious people who believe in heaven cannot fully be committed to human flourishing in this life, Hägglund claims. Only those who believe this life is all there is can live meaningfully here, fully committed to one another and the planet's flourishing.

Hägglund frequently describes this secular faith as having emancipatory potential, but it's anything but freeing. Rather it creates a paralyzing pressure: It's all on you! You have to make every moment—every second—matter. Time, after all, is the only thing that gives your life meaning.[9] What will you do while the clock ticks? Your fleeting little life means something only if you do significant things for others and for the planet as often as you can before you die, even if there's no ultimate framework for why any of it matters.

While some (like Bryan Johnson or Yuval Harari) respond to mortality by taking extreme measures to prolong life or pursue immortality, and others (like Hägglund) respond by committing to seize-your-moment activism on the basis of secular faith, both approaches—and all secular approaches—place a hopeless, crushing burden on the individual. Both approaches make life desperate and devoid of grace.

HOW CHRISTIANS SHOULD VIEW DEATH

Christians have a better framework for death. If sleep reminds believers of death—and it should!—it can point us to four truths.

1. Reminders of death provide eternal perspective. When believers follow contemporary culture's tendency to keep death out of sight and mind, we can start to live as if this life really is all that matters. The result is an earthly mindedness (Phil. 3:19) characterized by YOLO pressures to work through bucket lists and make your brief life mean something. But this is closer to Hägglund's secular faith than to Christian faith. As Cameron Cole argues in *Heavenward*, believers should lead lives in which "eternity organically and instinctively informs and drives the everyday matters of your life."[10] Sleep can be one of these organic reminders of eternity.

2. Awareness of mortality can make us wise. Whitney Pipkin says death "is a thousand commas strewn across our days reminding us that we, that those we love, that the world we inhabit, are all in a process of dying."[11] What are those commas? Cemeteries, migraines, falling leaves, rotten fruit, abandoned buildings, history museums, hospitals, canyons, comets, landfills, my rapidly graying beard, wrinkles on my forehead. Mortality is a fugue playing constantly on the pipe organ of the universe. "Sleep, sickness, weariness, and nighttime itself are ordinary and unbidden ashes on our foreheads," Tish Harrison Warren writes. "They say to us: remember that you are going to die."[12] But all these reminders aren't meant to make us morbid. Rather, the ashes all around are invitations to become wise. "Teach us to number our days, that we may gain a heart of wisdom" (Ps. 90:12). As Bobby Jamieson puts it, "Happiness comes not from denying or defying death but from letting death teach you humility."[13]

3. Eternity—not finitude—gives life urgency. Life is indeed a vapor (James 4:14). Christians are called to make the best use of their time (Eph. 5:16). Yet our urgency is driven not by the finitude of our lives but by the eternal destiny awaiting all people. If death can come for anyone at any moment, we should "make the most of every opportunity" (Col. 4:5) and do what we can to spread the gospel. Still, we ought to remember that our ultimate value has nothing to do with what we do for God but the fact that we belong to him. Our lives are not our own (1 Cor. 6:19). God made us, knows us, purposes our lives, keeps watch over our every movement. So as Christians, we can go to bed in peace, even if we feel frustratingly unproductive, having made little progress on our to-do lists. And we can approach our own deaths without anxiety that we didn't do everything, see everything, or make our lives count. This isn't the only life there is.

4. Death is still scary, sad, and worth mourning. Even though all of the above are true, it's okay for Christians to still find death scary. The after-death experience remains hauntingly unknown to us. And the unknown is scary. Even as we cling to trustworthy biblical assertions about death, resurrection, and the new creation, no one alive has ever experienced what it will be like. The mystery is unsettling. Furthermore, even though the sting of death has been removed by Christ's death and resurrection, death is still sad. It's right to mourn it (Eccl. 7:2), even as we mourn with hope (1 Thess. 4:13–14).

"I'LL SLEEP WHEN I'M DEAD"

Bon Jovi's 1992 song "I'll Sleep When I'm Dead" remains an appropriate anthem for our death-averse, no-time-to-waste modern world. The chorus declares, "Until I'm six feet under / Baby I don't need a bed / Gonna live while I'm alive / I'll sleep when I'm dead."

A pithy bit of rock-'n'-roll folk wisdom. A terrible ethos for life.

Sleep isn't a necessary evil to avoid so we can live more while we're alive. It's a grace that empowers living and prepares us for death, a theological mirror that nightly gives us a valuable image of our mortal frame. Mirrors don't always reflect an image we want to see. But they reflect the truth. And the truth, as Sufjan Stevens hauntingly repeats at the end of his song "Fourth of July," is this: "We're all gonna die."

Pause and Ponder

Pause

Right before bed some night this week—or on a regular basis as a bedtime ritual—read Psalm 90 and pray in response. Reflect on your mortality. Pray that God would use our nightly sleep as a constant reminder of the "sleep of death" to come (v. 5) and that this *memento mori* would "teach us to number our days" (v. 12).

Ponder

1. This chapter gives examples of how our culture tries to escape death, or at least hide it from view. Where else do you see this tendency in today's world or even in your own life?
2. In addition to leaning in to sleep's nightly reminder of our mortality, how else can we remember death in healthy ways that avoid our culture's desire to avoid or transcend it?
3. Euthanasia and physician-assisted suicide are increasingly normalized in modern Western culture, as part of a "right to die" movement that is gaining momentum. How is this a reflection of our desire for godlike control?
4. Even if Christians shouldn't fear death, why should we fight hard to preserve life even when a person is terminally ill or someone's life creates huge burdens for others?

4

BEST MEDICINE

We're Restored Through Rest

When we sleep we are not merely being released, we are also being restored. Without any effort of our own a new supply of energy is being built up within us.

—John Baíllíe, *Christian Devotion*

"I will refresh the weary and satisfy the faint."
At this I awoke and looked around. My sleep had been pleasant to me.

—Jeremiah 31:25–26

Wellness is all the rage. We're convinced that with the right cocktail of supplements, exercise, clean eating, and biometric monitoring (think smartwatches), we'll be on a path to peak humanity and a long life.

But what if the single most important thing we can do for "optimized health" is to do nothing for seven to eight hours each day? What if creation's most ingenious health hack is the regular rhythm of releasing our achievement drive and receiving a good night's sleep?

It's scandalous. It's offensive to our pride. How could something so passive, so indifferent to our willful efforts, be the miracle drug of our long-term health? But there's a growing consensus in the scientific and health communities that this is the case.

In God's wisdom, he created us such that we thrive most when we embrace regular stretches of ceased striving. The very thing ambitious people scoff at—"Sleep is for wimps!"[1]—is actually one of our greatest sources of strength.

What happens in our bodies and minds while we sleep is, quite simply, miraculous. Pretty much every "re-" word applies to what happens physically and mentally in sleep: regeneration, repair, restoration, recalibration, recuperation, rehabilitation. We all know the feeling of waking up after a great night's sleep and feeling renewed. Biologically it's almost as if after a solid sleep we are born again.

Christians have long appreciated the brilliance of God's design for sleep. In the third century, Tertullian wrote that "sleep is indispensable to our life, and health, and succour, there can be nothing pertaining to it which is not reasonable, and which is not natural."[2] God knew what he was doing when he created sleep and all the recalibrations it brings.

The extent of these recalibrations is becoming more known to science, and it's starting to shift the cultural conversation around sleep's importance. Scientists Steven Lockley and Russell Foster put it this way: "For centuries, we have regarded sleep as a simple suspension of activity, a passive state of unconsciousness, and for centuries we have been wrong. This failure to understand the active nature of sleep is perhaps one of the reasons why our 24-7 society has developed such little regard for it."[3]

It's time we listened to science on the active nature of sleep and spread the word as an act of neighbor love. For Christians, this is an opportunity to honor God with the stewardship of our bodies and glorify him for how "fearfully and wonderfully" we are made (Ps. 139:14).

WHAT SLEEP DOES FOR YOUR HEALTH

Prominent sleep researcher Matthew Walker describes sleep as "*the* universal health care provider: whatever the physical or mental ailment, sleep has a prescription it can dispense."[4] Details of sleep's many health benefits fill entire books (including Walker's). But in this chapter, I'll provide a short summary, organized around the two broad categories of physical and mental benefits.

PHYSICAL BENEFITS

Leave it to Shakespeare to poetically capture the multifaceted benefits of sleep. In *Macbeth*, the Bard sums it up:

> Sleep that knits up the raveled sleave of care,
> The death of each day's life, sore labor's bath,
> Balm of hurt minds, great nature's second course,
> Chief nourisher in life's feast.[5]

Shakespeare knew intuitively what modern science is proving empirically: Sleep really is the chief nourisher in life's feast. Some of the physical balms provided in sleep include:

- *Heart health.* Good sleep is closely tied to cardiovascular health. The heart keeps working during sleep, of course, but at a more restorative pace with a slower heart rate and lower blood pressure. Research shows good sleep correlates to better heart health and less likelihood of dying young.[6] One study showed that even sleeping in on the weekends—to compensate for less than ideal sleep during the work week—may lessen the risk of heart disease by up to 20 percent.[7]

- *Restored immune system.* Your mom was right. Sleep is the best medicine to heal sickness. "Sleep restocks the armory of our immune system,"[8] while insufficient sleep can make us more vulnerable to viruses and slow our recovery. Good sleep allows immune systems to release crucial proteins called cytokines to target infection or inflammation, as well as T cells to attack foreign viruses and bacteria.
- *Metabolism.* Good sleep helps regulate hormones, reduce inflammation, and promote a balanced microbiome in the gut, with healthy bacteria to aid food digestion and nutrient absorption. Sleep also releases proteins that suppress appetite and help maintain healthy weight.
- *Blood sugar.* Good sleep regulates our blood sugar and fine-tunes the balance of insulin and glucose in our system. Poor sleep—either too little or too much—has been associated with increased risk of diabetes.
- *Growth.* Kids grow in their sleep. The human growth hormone (HGH) is secreted by the pituitary gland largely at night, during deep sleep. Because no other demands are being made on the body physically during sleep, it is the opportune time for growth hormones to facilitate growth spurts. These hormones can cause a child to grow as much as two-thirds of an inch in twenty-four hours. In one study of infant growth, infants were shown to grow up to a tenth of an inch for every extra hour of sleep.[9]

MENTAL BENEFITS

In researching this book, I interviewed Mark Kohler, an Australian neuroscientist at the University of Adelaide and an evangelical Christian. Kohler has been doing sleep research for two decades and is currently focused on child sleep and cognition, sleep disorders, memory, and learning. Kohler sums up the scientific research on the benefits of sleep with the word *restoration*. All the research, he says, points to sleep's "restoring our cognitive capacity, restoring our emotional capacity, restoring of memories. . . . Sleep helps clear up the mess of the day."[10] Here are some ways sleep aids our cognitive flourishing:

"Offline" Memory and Information Processing

Our brains are very active in sleep: sorting, revising, and consolidating memories, filing away newly acquired experiences and learned skills. We'll look at this more in the next chapter, but scientists think dreaming is a byproduct of mental cataloging of the day's disparate inputs. "You take in information on your mental 'desk' during the day, and at night your brain tries to store it in various mental file cabinets," Kohler says. "If the brain does this right, retrieval of that information through memory is easier at a later stage." Another pair of sleep researchers claims, "For every two hours we spend awake, storing away new information, our brain needs an hour of sleep to figure out the meaning and significance of that new information."[11] And it needs to do this work in a focused state, disconnected from the outside world and with our normal inputs and waking-life governance turned off. This function is so critical that some scientists point to "sleep-dependent memory processing" as one of the most compelling theories for the necessity of sleep.[12]

Understanding the World

Sleep is a time when the brain catches up with the day's onslaught of inputs, discovering patterns and rules about how the world works and who we are within it. This is one reason why infants need *so much* sleep. They are constantly learning, taking in the novel world for the first time. Unlike adults, they can't wait all day for nighttime sleep to store and process all this newly acquired information. "Without periodic naps to allow their sleeping brains to process the new information their little brains are taking in, they get overloaded," Antonio Zadra and Robert Stickgold argue. "They start feeling burned out and crabby, just like adults who have taken in too much information without a break."[13]

Creativity and Problem Solving

Good sleep can result in cracking difficult conundrums or coming to a creative epiphany. (Paul McCartney claimed "Yesterday" and "Let It Be" came to him in his sleep.) As we sleep, our brains work without our conscious participation to creatively solve problems. There's a reason the colloquial phrase "sleep on it" exists in most languages and cultures around the world. Much of what we call dreaming is this "informational alchemy" wherein the brain "tests out and builds connections between vast stores of information . . . [i]n ways your waking brain would never attempt."[14]

I find this mind-blowing. What's not obvious to us in the light of day—the problems we can't solve, the big decisions we're struggling to make—can become clearer in the morning because of how our brains make sense of things while we sleep. Matthew Walker goes so far as to describe the brain's deep nocturnal work as "the difference between knowledge (retention of individual facts) and wisdom (knowing what they all mean when you fit them together)."[15]

As we sleep, our fragmentary thoughts become integrated and more coherent. We become wiser. What a marvelous Creator!

Mental and Emotional Health

Sleep can also do wonders for us emotionally. Quality sleep is associated with improved mood, reduced stress, and overall psychological health. It reduces stress and can help with anxiety and depression. Lack of sleep does the opposite. When we observe that a grump "woke up on the wrong side of bed," it's possibly an outcome of less than ideal sleep.

Dreaming sleep in particular plays a mysterious role in emotional healing. Walker calls it a form of "overnight therapy" that "takes the painful sting out of difficult, even traumatic, emotional episodes you have experienced during the day, offering emotional resolution when you awake the next morning."[16] Elsewhere he describes REM dreaming as "a consoling neurochemical bath that mollifies painful memories" and provides healing: "To sleep, perchance to heal."[17]

When we go to bed in emotional turmoil, often (though not always) a good night's sleep will leave us feeling less distraught and a bit more recalibrated. John Baíllíe observed this in a 1957 sermon on sleep: "Our minds are clearer, and very often we find that the problems of the day before have settled themselves while we slept."[18]

How remarkable that God, in his kindness, created a mechanism not just for physical restoration as we sleep but also for emotional restoration.

Keeping Time

Though keeping time is not necessarily a restorative cognitive benefit, it's still quite amazing. Do you ever set your alarm before you go to bed, knowing you have to get up at, say, 5:00 a.m., and then your body mysteriously wakes up at 4:59 a.m. even without the help of the alarm clock ring? This is because your brain "is still capable of logging time with quite remarkable precision while asleep."[19] Unreal! And this is just one of many fascinating health benefits tied to the body's "master clock" circadian rhythm. Mark Kohler told me, "Our bodies' circadian rhythm (the master clock) also consists of multiple peripheral clocks found throughout the body and which work together to regulate daily rhythms in physiology, behavior, and metabolism. There are peripheral clocks in nearly all tissues and organs, including our liver, heart, and gut. Just like the master clock is sensitive to light, peripheral clocks are sensitive to other non-light cues such as the timing of food intake (when you eat), physical activity, and temperature. For optimal health (mental and physical) we want our sleep-timing, central, and peripheral clocks to be synchronized with each other and with the external environment."

HEALTH DANGERS OF LACK OF SLEEP

As much as the benefits of good sleep have become clearer, so too have the ominous costs of poor sleep. As one expert put it, "Without sleep, we would soon die, and without good sleep, we will die sooner."[20] Consider this nonexhaustive list of how health can go awry as a result of poor sleep:

Short-Term

- Moodiness, stress, anxiety, irritability
- Weaker immunity to ward off or recover from sickness
- Impaired cognition, trouble concentrating, forgetfulness
- Drowsiness (especially dangerous when driving)
- Poorer school or athletic performance

Long-Term

- Decreased growth-hormone (GH) levels, affecting muscle mass, bone density, energy levels, and more
- Increased risk of cardiovascular disease,[21] metabolic disorders and diabetes, and certain forms of cancer
- Increased risk of developing Alzheimer's disease or dementia
- Weight gain[22]
- Higher blood pressure
- Increased risk of stroke
- Poorer cognitive and motor function
- Reproductive harm for men, including lower sperm counts and lower testosterone[23]

If we get into the habit of sleeping less than we should, our lifespans likely will be shorter. Insufficient sleep has been linked to seven of fifteen leading causes of death in the United States. For Christians, it's time to stop viewing sleep as wasteful, or minimizing its value as a nice-to-have. Sleep is a crucial part of stewarding the bodies God gave us. To value sleep is to be pro-life.

SLEEP DISORDERS AND THE PAIN OF NONRESTORATIVE SLEEP

You might be thinking, "I know the importance of this, and I try to get good sleep each night. But I can't." I hear you. You're not alone. In the US, more than fifty million people suffer from at least one sleep disorder. Common disorders include insomnia, narcolepsy, sleep apnea, restless leg syndrome, somnambulism (sleepwalking), and the truly scary fatal familial insomnia (discussed in depth in chapter 10).

The reality in our fallen world is that good gifts are marred. God's creation, though perfect in its original design, is now in bondage to decay, groaning for restoration and liberation (Rom. 8:19–22). Sleep is one of the best gifts we have, but it's rarely perfect. For some sufferers, it's rarely even good. The "groaning" of sleep speaks to our sure hope of eternal rest. Deeply restorative rest is hard to come by in the *now*. But we'll experience it in the *not yet*. The present imperfection of sleep should inflame our hearts to long for the perfect rest to come.

This is only partial consolation, however, for those suffering through restless nights, aching for replenishing sleep. What can you do *now* to overcome sleep challenges? For one, you should talk to a doctor and get medical help. Great advances are being made in the field of sleep disorders, and treatments and medications can alleviate some of your pain. As we've seen, solving the problem of poor sleep now will likely preemptively solve a bevy of other health problems down the road. So seek medical health!

Also, pray. I know friends with sleep disorders who were healed or found significant relief after diligently asking for healing prayers. God is a healer, and we know he delights in giving his beloved sleep (Ps. 127:2). Ask him for it. Weep and groan to him.

TIPS FOR GETTING GOOD SLEEP

Whether or not you struggle to sleep, most of us could use more of it. Almost 35 percent of US adults fail to get the recommended seven hours of nightly sleep. Other developed countries are even worse. (UK: 39 percent; Japan: 66 percent.)[24] Globally, sleep deficiency is a health epidemic. The downstream effects are severe.

Thankfully, there are a number of minor tweaks we can make to set ourselves up for better sleep. Here are a few:

- *Stick to a schedule.* Routine is one of the best aids for good sleep. Go to bed and get up at roughly the same time each day. This helps sync your body to a predictable sleep-wake cycle that leads to better, deeper sleep. Plan your bedtime to ensure seven to eight hours of sleep each night—not much less or much more.
- *Sleep in darkness.* Our bodies are designed to get sleep when night's darkness sets in. The natural trigger of sunset has now been replaced by ubiquitous artificial lights that can brighten our rooms—or glow from a device screen—at all hours of the night. Get ready for bed by dimming lights. (Maybe read in bed with only a small reading lamp at your bedside.) Then sleep in total darkness, ideally with room-darkening shades.
- *Sleep in cooler temperatures.* Our bodies are also designed to sleep when temperatures drop, again following the natural cycle of night bringing colder temperatures. But climate-controlled dwellings can now maintain the same temperature throughout the day and night, which goes against the grain of our design. Address this by turning down your thermostat when you go to bed, ideally to between 65 and 68 degrees F (or 18 to 20 degrees C). Your body sleeps better in cooler temperatures.
- *Avoid caffeine, nicotine, and alcohol before bed.* For at least several hours prior to bedtime, avoid these proven disruptors of good sleep.
- *Exercise during the day (but not too late in the day).* Being physically active during the day can help you fall asleep faster and tends to improve overall sleep quality. Vigorous physical activity too close to bedtime, however, may delay your ability to fall to sleep easily.
- *No screens before bed!* This is a common culprit behind modern sleep woes. Most of us try to wind down right before bed

by scrolling or streaming on screens. Don't! It's not just the light from screens that's problematic; it's the mental stress of going to bed with a last-minute avalanche of fragmented, often troubling information. Doomscrolling before bed—really any scrolling before bed—is a bad idea. If you need media to chill out before bed, read a physical book.

NEW LIFE FROM THE DEATH OF SLEEP

The more we learn about sleep science, the more Christians should marvel at the goodness of God and the wonders of his creation. Mark Kohler says he's constantly fascinated with God's design in creation, of which sleep is "up there among the most amazing." Kohler thinks sleep points to a God of order, who puts everything in balance and wants us to rest in him—and be restored.

Still, sleep can feel to us like a little death. To lie down at night and turn off for eight hours requires humility and trust. But the more we know about how God designed sleep to restore us—physically and mentally—the more we grasp how this deathlike posture is in fact a vibrant venue in which God renews our lives. Yet as in our spiritual renewal, this bodily renewal requires us to relax our fierce will—to loosen our grip and let God do his work. John Baíllíe beautifully draws out the spiritual implications of this physical reality:

> During the day we are so anxious to keep the reins of our destiny so entirely in our own hands that God has to wait until we are asleep in order to do for us and in us those things which we cannot do for ourselves. . . . If some of the processes that are necessary for our physical well-being go on more advantageously

> in sleep than in waking life, because the will then relaxes its too despotic control, why should not the same be true of some of the processes that advance our spiritual well-being?[25]

So don't fear the "death of each day's life." Rather, rejoice in the nocturnal balm God created for you, to heal your hurt mind and restore your weary body. Sleep in a state of trust, as Wendell Berry describes poetically:

> However heart or head may ache;
> I go to sleep when I lie down.
> With no determined care to breathe,
> I breathe and live and sleep and take.[26]

We don't will the wonders that occur in sleep ("with no determined care"). But we gladly take them. As in faith we receive God's grace—a gift of God, not by works (Eph. 2:8–9)—so in faith we turn off the lights, turn down the thermostat, pull up the covers, and surrender to sleep's gracious convalescence.

Pause and Ponder

Pause

Audit your sleep quality. Are you getting seven or more hours of sleep at night? If not, what can you do to set yourself up for better sleep? Even within the limitations of your particular situation (late-night or early-morning work hours, parenting infants, or something else), consider how you might implement some of the tips for getting better sleep listed in this chapter. If you struggle with (or believe you might have) a sleep disorder that has not yet been addressed, consider reaching out to a healthcare provider to see what options exist for addressing it.

Ponder

1. What is one thing you learned in this chapter that you can start implementing in the hope of getting better sleep?
2. What does it mean theologically that sleep—an action that is really a surrender to receive—brings such profound life and vitality to our holistic health?
3. If you have struggled with poor sleep in the past but found solutions that improved your sleep quality, share these tips with others! If you're discussing this book in a group setting, spend a few minutes sharing the best practices and habits that have helped you sleep better.

5

PERCHANCE TO DREAM

We're Made to Imagine

Even a soul submerged in sleep is hard at work
and helps make something of the world.
—Heraclitus, *Fragments*

I had a dream that made me afraid. As I was
lying in bed, the images and visions that
passed through my mind terrified me.
—Daniel 4:5

As a kid I designed roller coasters in my mind as I drifted off to sleep. And elaborate floor plans for houses. For a season I spent this meandering reverie time envisioning the New Jerusalem's architectural wonders (twelve gates, massive cube shape), wondering whether it might include Disneyland-style monorails or Wonka-style magic elevators. All in my mind. All in the few minutes between lying down in bed and falling asleep.

Human consciousness is mind-blowing. We have the capacity to imagine entire worlds and go there without ever moving an inch. We create mental experiences that can feel so real.

It's supernatural. Our ability to imagine things that don't exist is a way we imitate our creator God, who spoke the universe into being *ex nihilo*. "The imagination of man is made in the image of the imagination of God," George MacDonald once said.[1] To be sure, our imagination is also unlike God's. We don't imagine things *ex nihilo*; our imagination is constrained by the raw materials of what we've already perceived. Yet our capacity to remix reality and imagine something new—some previously unthought thought, undreamt possibility, undiscovered innovation—is still miraculous and a powerful way the image of God in us is evident.

Our imagination is highly active in waking life. But it works in overdrive while we sleep. For seven or more hours a night, we dream—a very small fraction of it remembered when we wake, most of it forgotten. Why did God create our imaginative minds to be so active while we sleep? What is dreaming's purpose?

It's a big, fascinating question that has piqued human curiosity from time immemorial. In this chapter I'll summarize some of the answers contemporary science offers, theories of the biological utility of dreaming. Then in chapter 6, I'll reflect on how Christianity gives us additional categories for considering the point of dreams.

Buckle up. This was the most mind-blowing chapter of the book for me to research and write. I hope you'll be as mentally and spiritually stimulated as I was, provoked to worship the awesome God who created our dreaming capacity and is sovereign over it.

WHAT IS DREAMING?

What *is* dreaming? History is full of ideas, including Freud's prominent psychological theory (now largely dismissed by the scientific community) that dreams are a sort of relief valve for repressed desires. But since the discovery of rapid eye movement (REM) sleep in the 1950s, the biological understanding of dreams has greatly advanced.

Dream researchers Antonio Zadra and Robert Stickgold define dreams as "any mental experience that occurs during sleep—any thoughts, feelings, or images that come into our awareness while we sleep."[2] Rapid eye movement sleep—"a unique body state that is not seen at any other time of the day or night"[3]—happens about every ninety minutes, across the entire sleep period. Between these REM sleeps are other distinct, non-REM (NREM) stages—N1, N2, and N3—which each represent a deeper descent into dreaming consciousness. Rapid eye movement is so named because we can observe it physically in those who are in this sleep stage. (If you've ever watched a baby's eyes in REM sleep, you know what it looks like.) A leading theory of what's happening physically is the "scanning hypothesis," which proposes that the brain tracks the action in our dreams with the physical gaze direction of our eyes.

We likely dream throughout the night, with different types of dreams at each stage. REM dreaming is the climax and often involves vivid imagery, structured but often unusual scenarios, and intense emotions. It's associated with higher breathing and heart rates and more blood flow to the brain.[4] During REM our brains are very active (EEGs show electrical activity on par with what we see in wakeful states), even as bodily movements are suppressed, leaving us with limited ability to control our muscles (called "atonia"). Without this crucial suppression of physical activity, our muscles would want to act out our dreams and respond physically to the mental stimulation in them. Yikes!

During REM sleep, certain parts of the brain are selectively activated or deactivated. Emotional parts are activated, while the parts underlying logical reasoning and reflective thought are deactivated. This is why our dreams often feel deeply emotional, but wildly illogical.[5] Dream research has shown interesting commonalities in dream content, with the most commonly reported dreams in both men and women involving themes of being chased, sexual experiences, school, teachers, studying, and falling.[6] Even though scientists think we dream multiple times every night, the average adult remembers only four to six dreams per month, and even those are typically soon forgotten. So "whatever the function of dreams may be, it simply cannot depend on our remembering them once we awaken."[7]

SCIENCE'S TAKE ON DREAMING

If dreaming only occasionally has overlap with our waking consciousness (via infrequently half-remembered dreams), what is the function of dreaming? Why would God create us with this function that plays out roughly a third of our lives as we sleep? Or as evolutionary scientists would put it, what is the biological-utilitarian purpose dreaming serves, explaining why humans are such avid nocturnal dreamers? The following three metaphors provide some examples of current ways scientists are answering this question.

1. DIGESTION

Just as the food we take in goes through a necessary process of digestion that sifts through nutrients to keep and waste to eliminate, so too do our mental inputs. The dreaming brain is sorting through cognitive inputs, trying to discern what to absorb and what to discard.

One thing Freud was right about is his concept of "day residue": Our dream content incorporates bits and pieces of experiences, emotions, and other mental intakes from the previous day. But "rather than incorporating an entire episodic memory from the preceding day's events, our brain takes only pieces of them: objects, settings, people, impressions, fleeting thoughts, or bits of conversations."[8] These bits of day residue then get combined—in ways that feel random and jarring, hence the bizarreness of our dreams—with older memories from weeks or years earlier. In dreaming, the brain is trying to figure out what new material is important to keep and what existing category of memories it fits within or connects to.

My Christian neuroscientist friend, Mark Kohler, puts it this way: "Dreaming is not just about making discrete memories of single pieces of information; it's about making links and connections. How does this bit of information relate to the broader topic I've learned about? How does this experience remind me of or relate to other experiences I've had?" This helps explain why dreams so often prompt psychoanalytic interpretations, Kohler says. "You're dreaming these things because they are representations not just of discrete events but also of your brain's interpretation of those events, which probably relies on or relates to other experiences you've had in life."

Why must this mental digestion happen while we sleep? Scientists suspect dreaming's sleep-dependency has to do with the brain needing undistracted time to "reorder the information inside our heads, to get rid of certain obsolete memories, to update memories, and to incorporate new experiences into our memory systems."[9] During the day, we accumulate huge amounts of sensorimotor and emotional data, but the requirements of waking life mean our brains can't multitask and digest this data simultaneously. The crucial processing task is reserved for sleep, when the brain at last has space for the deep work of organizing information.

As I mentioned in the previous chapter, this is one reason babies need so much sleep. It's not just that their little bodies get physically tired sooner. Their brains get exhausted sooner and can't wait all day for the mental digestion to begin. They need to sleep more often to keep pace with the buffet of new cognitive food—spatial skills, language, images perceived for the first time—they're constantly consuming. So if you're wondering whether babies dream, the answer is yes! They actually dream (have REM sleep) more in their first few months of life than at any other stage of development. The content of baby dreams is impossible to know, however. (Obviously researchers can't interview babies or prompt them to record dream reports.) Whatever babies dream about would have to be limited to their nascent, preverbal consciousness and basic knowledge and skills they've attained—perhaps "little more than a pastiche of remembered sensations and emotions."[10]

2. ARTIST'S STUDIO

Scientists also think dreaming is like a creative workspace. Any artist will tell you they need dedicated space—away from everyday distractions and tasks—for creative inspiration. Creativity requires good inputs, but also focused time and space for these inputs to be turned into original outputs.

Nocturnal dreaming is like the writer's cabin in the woods, the painter's seaside cottage, the musician's studio: set-apart places where we can take the raw materials of life and imaginatively remix them into new visions, new possibilities, new interpretations. Dreaming is a vital place where ideas can percolate, possibilities can emerge, connections can be forged, rough sketches can be attempted, all with waking-life implications for how we live.

Zadra and Stickgold use the artist metaphor to summarize their theory of dreaming: The dreaming brain "attempts only to show us what has been and what might be. It does so in the same way as a great painter or composer, novelist, or playwright might—by *showing* us what we cannot yet fully explain. Arguably, that is the function of art; and we believe it is also the function of dreaming."[11]

Scientists have discovered that REM sleep fuels creativity and can spark epiphanies, novel solutions, and creative breakthroughs in waking life. In particular, dreams can help us solve problems that require outside-the-box thinking. As one researcher put it, "When we are stuck on a problem, dreams can supply the breakthrough."[12] Matthew Walker notes that Dmitri Mendeleev came up with the periodic table of elements after waking up one morning: "As he slept, he dreamed, and his dreaming brain accomplished what his waking brain was incapable of."[13]

When I speak to aspiring writers, one thing I talk about is the importance of three elements in every great creative endeavor: nourishing inputs, time and space to process those inputs, and finally turning those inputs into an output you offer to the world. It's stunning how much in God's creation is defined by this three-part cycle (inputs, processing, outputs).

Think of the seed-to-plant cycle. Inputs of sunlight and water are required first, followed by processing time—seed dormancy, germination, growth—before the outputs of sprouts, buds, leaves, or fruit. It's the same recipe for human and animal multiplication: inputs (father's sperm, mother's egg) + processing time (gestation in the mother's womb) + output (birth into the world as a new being, distinct from the inputs that made it). We see an echo of this cycle even in the death and resurrection of our Savior: the input of his Good Friday death and burial, the processing time of Sabbath, and the explosive, world-altering output of his Easter resurrection. Our dreaming time is a bit like Holy Saturday—a mysterious liminal space between the often-painful inputs of Friday and the new life of Sunday.

Between the darkness of night and the brightness of day, our dreaming brains can process and remake the world.

It seems God values the time between inputs and outputs. He could have created trees to sprout instantly after the inputs of sun and rain, babies to be born the next day after being conceived. He didn't. He's an unhurried God who values process (sometimes longer than we like!) over instant results.[14] The creative breathing room of our dreaming sleep shows that he wants our lives to be marked by process too.

3. TRIP PLANNING

I have a geeky obsession with trip planning: exploring possibilities, constructing itineraries, and making plans for future family ventures.

There's no shortage of inputs available for this: travel apps, TripAdvisor reviews, AI-generated sample itineraries. Google "how to spend three days in Barcelona" and copious suggestions surface. Yet like anything else in life, you can't go directly from an overwhelming array of inputs to a coherent output. That's why I don't recommend waiting until the day before you leave on a trip to start researching. You need time to cull the information, notice patterns of overlapping tips, make connections with your experiences, and "try out" various permutations of itineraries: where to go and what to do, for how long. You need time to envision and experiment with the future and make mental maps of where you're going and what you'll do.

Dreaming is sort of like this. It involves mental mapping and future-priming exploration of possibilities. In *When Brains Dream*, Antonio Zadra and Robert Stickgold advocate for an explanatory theory of dreaming they call NEXTUP (network exploration to understand possibilities): "You can think of it as similar to the true goal of education—not to cram facts into our brains, but rather to open us to the unexplored possibilities embodied within those facts, showing us the many ways they can be used and not just one specific way."[15]

The phrase "true goal of education" is helpful because it hints at the folly of trying only to accumulate inputs without leaving space for processing those inputs. Dreaming is not just about the facts your brain has collected. It's about making sense of them, connecting the dots (often in unexpected ways), bringing experience to bear on new information, and putting everything together in a way that better prepares you for the future.

The secret sauce of the planning that occurs in dreams is that there is risk-free, experimental freedom to consider wild possibilities and search "more widely than during wakefulness, going through less obvious associations, and digging for hidden treasures in places it would never consider while awake."[16] Our waking brains will often chastise us for thinking of some outlandish idea: "That's a silly idea! That could never happen." But our dreaming brains have no problem swinging for the fences with bold, seemingly illogical or unlikely possibilities.

Every year, I come up with two or three summer trip ideas for our family, spending a decent amount of time putting together sample itineraries for each. Usually there's a crazier option in the mix (two weeks in Canada with three kids under six!) and a few more reasonable ideas (rent an Airbnb near a US national park for a week). I pitch these options to my wife, Kira, around February each year and see how she reacts. I suspect she'll opt for the more conservative option, but I present all options because—who knows?—she might actually go for the reach idea. And it might end up being a trip of a lifetime for our family! Many great experiences start as ideas that at first feel outrageous.

This is akin to what the NEXTUP dreaming theory suggests: We dream to consider all options and permutations, to play out all scenarios, and to prepare ourselves for possible futures, especially ones our rational waking selves might never consider.

Dreaming helps us picture ourselves in different worlds, bringing the future to us before we experience it. This is what I do in trip planning when I'm looking at Google maps of Paris and crafting a logical walking route or picturing my family on a hike after reading a trail summary and seeing pictures online. The research inputs help me construct mental images of a future reality, allowing me to walk in the shoes of future treks and mentally picture what might be.

Similarly, in our dreams our brains create "an amazingly comprehensive virtual world" in which we "can partake every night of a world with literally endless possibilities."[17] All without moving from our beds.

OUR MARVELOUS MAKER

If this were all we knew about how dreams serve human flourishing, it would be more than enough for us to gratefully praise our Creator. How gratuitously loving of him to build into our brains these astonishing capacities:

- To nightly process newly acquired information, skills, memories, emotions

- To organize and interpret these inputs, making connections we'd never think to make in waking life
- To creatively play around with new ideas
- To envision and prepare for various possibilities

All in our sleep. All while our other bodily systems are doing their own recalibrations. All without our willful involvement! How wonderful. How marvelous.

And yet as Christians, we know there's even more to say about dreaming. Dreams figure prominently in Scripture and Christian tradition, and our faith brings a whole other dimension to our understanding of dreams. The topic of dreams is a perfect example of where the two books of revelation (Scripture and nature) really can help paint a fuller, more majestic picture of reality. We've just summarized what the second book has to say. Let's now consider dreams through the lens of the first book.

Pause and Ponder

Pause

The next time you wake up with a dream still lingering in memory with some clarity, write down as much of its narrative details as you can remember. Then look over what you wrote and consider what inputs (either from the previous day or from longer ago) might have been the source material for the dream. See how much you can trace from what the dream was about and what mental inputs from real life may have precipitated it.

Ponder

1. Which of the three scientific metaphors for dreaming's purpose do you find most fascinating? What is the most interesting thing you learned about dreaming in this chapter?
2. Have you ever experienced going to sleep thinking about a complex problem or decision, only to wake up in the morning with sudden clarity or peace?
3. If one of the key functions of dreams is to give our minds undistracted time to process mental inputs, what does this say about God's valuing of process over efficiency?
4. We experience REM dreaming sleep for most of the night, every night of our lives, but we remember only a tiny fraction of our dreams—and even the ones we remember typically fade quickly. Why do you think God created us to forget the vast majority of our dreams?

6

ONLY A DREAM?

We're Made to Receive

Seek not that your sons and your daughters should not see visions, should not dream dreams; seek that they should see true visions, that they should dream noble dreams.
—George MacDonald, "The Imagination: Its Function and Its Culture"

Then Solomon awoke—and he realized it had been a dream.
—1 Kings 3:15

Dreams loom large in Scripture. They frequently figure into God's plans in history, catalyzing key events often in dramatic ways. If we believe anything in God's Word, we have to believe he sovereignly uses human dreams to advance his purposes. He moves people, convicts sinners, catalyzes missional action, and more through this state of altered consciousness that we cannot control but can only receive.

The meandering, often harrowing phantasmagoria of dreams isn't always life-altering or meaningful. (We immediately forget the vast majority of them, after all.) But sometimes it is. And this is not just biblically clear. It's experientially clear in the everyday lives of people throughout history—even today. Even for the irreligious, the experience of dreaming often feels supernatural—a mystical realm wherein something beyond my individual consciousness is at work. But for Christians, we need not grasp after an inexplicable something shaping our dreams. We know there is a sovereign someone with a track record of molding human dreams for his purposes. In this chapter we'll ponder a bit of what that looks like.

SCRIPTURE'S TAKE ON DREAMING

In the previous chapter we explored three general-revelation metaphors for what's happening biologically in our dreams (by God's design). In this chapter we'll add three special-revelation metaphors that help us see what's going on spiritually in our dreams.

1. DIVINE COMMUNICATION

Dreams are a way God communicates with people for a variety of reasons (Job 33:14–18): warning, comforting, convicting, explaining, preserving, and giving foreknowledge. God himself says he communicates this way (Num. 12:6). And he demonstrates it frequently:

- Jacob's dream at Bethel (Gen. 28:10–22), which reassures him of God's presence, protection, and promises
- Joseph's dreams and interpretations of dreams in Genesis (37:1–11; 40–41), which contribute to his rise in a pagan ruler's court

- Solomon's dream at Gibeon (1 Kings 3:5–15), in which he asks God for wisdom and God grants it
- Daniel's dreams (Daniel 7) and interpretations of Nebuchadnezzar's dreams (Daniel 2, 4), which—like Joseph—propel him to prominence in a pagan court
- Joseph's dreams (Matt. 1:20–21; 2:13, 19–22) confirming who Jesus is and how Joseph can protect him from the murderous Herod
- Pilate's wife's dream (Matt. 27:19), which leads her to try to convince her husband to release Jesus
- Paul's dream of a man of Macedonia (Acts 16:9–10), which prompts him to go immediately to Macedonia to preach the gospel

These and other examples show that God is sovereign over dreams, including the dreams of pagans. Pilate's wife's dream is especially fascinating because the action it catalyzes (her desire to release Jesus) does not come to pass. Historians aren't sure what happened to her after this. But if she went on to become a Christian, maybe this dream was God's way of pricking her conscience and convincing her Jesus is Lord.

Sometimes God uses dreams to catalyze big things in history. Other times he uses dreams to change one life.

Examples abound in church history. Early church father Jerome, who translated the Bible into Latin, points to a dream as a catalyst for his decisive shift toward reading God's Word with greater zeal than he read the classics of men. (The dream is visually depicted in Matteo di Giovanni's 1476 painting *The Dream of Saint Jerome*.) Dreams were pivotal in Saint Patrick's life, both in leading him to escape slavery in Ireland and then later in prompting him to return to Ireland to bring the Christian gospel to the Celtic pagan land. When he was a rebellious teenage sailor, "Amazing Grace" hymn writer John Newton had an impressionable yet peculiar dream about a ring. Years later he recalled the dream at a pivotal point in his spiritual journey, and it led him to a profound trust in God's sovereignty: "O what an unspeakable comfort is this, that I am not in my own keeping!"[1]

God uses dreams to stir souls and advance his mission even today. A big example of this is how central dreams are in the surging growth of Christianity in the Middle East. One recent report on Muslim converts to Christianity showed that a quarter experienced a dream that led to their conversion—often a dream in which Jesus appeared and spoke Scripture to them, sometimes Scripture they had never heard before.[2]

As Mark Kohler reminded me, in a lot of cultures, "dreaming is such a normal way of hearing things spiritually."[3] Modern Western cultures tend to be more skeptical of the idea of dreams as divine communication, but even here it's not hard to find people who've had at least one dream experience they'd categorize as supernatural: prophetic, revelatory, or somehow charged with the divine.

I belong to a Reformed-charismatic church network. It's common to have people in our tribe share dreams they feel God gave them as a message for a particular church or an individual member. I've witnessed several occasions when someone's dream played a pivotal role in building up our church body, including one dream that led to the location where our church plant met its first three years. My wife, Kira, has occasionally had dreams about people she hadn't talked to or seen in years, but they left such an impression that she felt prompted to reach out and check in. In every instance, the timing of the reconnection proved profound—a "divine appointment."

God still speaks through dreams. We're still in the last-days age of the church, in which "your sons and daughters will prophesy, your young men will see visions, your old men will dream dreams"

(Acts 2:17–18). Even if you're not part of a charismatic tradition, be open to the idea that God might use your dreams to convict, confirm, or nudge you in a certain direction. Pay special attention to the dreams you remember when you wake up, dreams that linger in your memory. Jot them down in a dream journal. See whether you notice patterns over time. Is God trying to get your attention? If you're facing a big decision, pray God might give clarity or confirmation through dreams—either yours or the dreams of others.

2. HAUNTED HOUSE

Sometimes dreams feel like haunted houses, with terrors behind every turn and no clear exit. Dreams in which you're trying to run but can't move. Dreams in which you open your mouth but can't scream. Dreams of a scary bogeyman you see in the distance, who spots you and then starts walking directly toward you. (I dreamed this as a kid, and the image still haunts me.)

Dreaming has a dark side.

Nightmares are a universal feature of human dreaming. Approximately 85 percent of adults report having at least one bad dream per year. About a quarter of US adults have had an experience of sleep paralysis too—the terrifying sleep disorder where REM-induced muscle paralysis continues after you wake, often combined with dreamlike hallucinations that occur while your waking eyes are wide open.

While scientists explain sleep paralysis as simply a dream-related dysfunction, sufferers of it can't shake the feeling that it's supernatural. Many report the felt experience of an oppressive presence in the room or on their bodies in a suffocating way. Some describe these bedroom visitors as shadowy figures, aliens, or demons. In the disturbing documentary *The Nightmare*, one woman describes her sleep paralysis experiences as "a kind of horror that is worse than what is in the movies. It's an icy cold, kind of dark, evil, something's in the room and it's watching me. . . . It wants you to feel afraid."[4]

Christians have language for experiences that feel viscerally demonic: spiritual warfare. Just as dreams can be arenas where God meets us and speaks to us, they can also be opportunities for the devil to gain a foothold—particularly in seasons of heightened stress, emotional turmoil, or other spiritual vulnerabilities. Tertullian thought dreams could be communication from God *or* demons. Satan, he wrote, "never withdraws his malignant efforts to steal over [Christians] as best he may in their very sleep, if unable to assault them when they are awake."[5]

3. HALL OF MIRRORS

Our dreams are scary not only because demons can lurk in their shadowy rooms but also because sometimes we're in a hall of mirrors where the horror isn't an external evil but rather some uncomfortable aspect of ourselves reflected back to us. There's a moral-mirroring aspect to our dreams that can be troubling, but instructive. Gregory of Nyssa observed this back in the fourth century:

> Most men's dreams are conformed to the state of their character: the brave man's fancies are of one kind, the coward's of another; the wanton man's dreams of one kind, the continent man's of another; the liberal man and the avaricious man are subject to different fancies; while these fancies are nowhere framed by the intellect, but by the less rational disposition of the soul, which forms even in dreams the semblances of those things to which each is accustomed by the practice of his waking hours.[6]

Gregory's saying what we all have experienced: Our dreams often reflect our longings from waking life, and these reflections are sometimes disconcerting and ugly. We often do things in our dreams we would never do in waking life. With the rational part of our brains turned off, our emotions and desires can meander down dark paths, often in the genre of illicit sexual acts. The experience—if we remember the dream—can leave us feeling guilty and concerned: Why would I dream such an abominable thing?

What should we make of these situations? On one hand we can remind ourselves that we can't rationally resist temptation as easily in dreams as we can in waking life. Augustine, in *Confessions*, said, "I return to a clear conscience when I wake and realize . . . I was not responsible for the act, although I am sorry that by some means or other it happened to me."[7] Still, it can be frustrating to battle sexual temptation ardently in daytime, only to seemingly indulge it in dreams.

John Piper responds to this common burden in an *Ask Pastor John* podcast episode. On one hand, he notes (citing Isa. 29:7–8) that "there is nothing remarkable" when a physical craving like hunger or thirst or sexual desire causes us to have dreams where those cravings are satisfied. Dreams reveal real desires, which are sometimes desires disordered by sinful nature. Maybe the devil can use this desire-fueled dream content to shame and accuse us. But God can also use these dreams to test our faith and warn us. Piper says the question is less why you're dreaming these things and more what you'll do in response, in waking life: "Will the dream have its God-appointed effect of humbling us, frightening us about our own bent to sinning? And will we lay hold on him for purity in waking life?"[8]

Morally dark dreams are troubling, especially when we are the one in the dream who is engaging in some immoral act. We ought to respond with a newfound fervor for holiness, knowing that God might be prodding our consciences in a sanctifying way. But are there ways we might avoid the darker content of dreams altogether, or at least reduce its frequency? Are dreams totally out of our control, or are there habits that can lead to less troubling dreams? As we conclude this chapter, let's ponder this practical question.

CAN—AND SHOULD—WE CONTROL OUR DREAMS?

Lucid dreaming is all the rage. In a biohacking age when we seek to control and optimize everything—even the uncontrolled space of sleep—perhaps this is not surprising. But is it wise?

In its broadest definition, lucid dreaming is simply anytime you're aware you are dreaming as you dream.[9] It can be a comforting relief when, in the midst of a troubling dream, you become aware that it's just a dream. In more extreme forms, lucid dreaming becomes a developed skill where the dreamer consciously dictates aspects of their behavior in a dream narrative—a phenomenon that sounds like science fiction but has been confirmed through laboratory studies.[10]

Because there is big money to be made in lucid dreaming—as part of the booming wellness business—technologies and treatments are rapidly being developed. Certainly there will be helpful uses for it, especially for those who suffer from nightmares and dream-related sleep disorders. A recent Northwestern University study, for example, showed that a method called targeted lucidity reactivation (TLR) helped reduce narcolepsy-related nightmares in six patients. The study involved the patients "rewriting" their nightmares into more pleasant dreams, then "rehearsing" the new scripts before falling asleep each night.[11]

But I don't think we should obsessively try to hack our dreams via new apps, how-to books, and lucid-dreaming devices. Some realms, like our sleep, are uncontrollable by God's design. We'd do well to minimize our interference. Still, the basic premise of lucid dreaming feels like common sense: What you think about as you fall asleep can influence what you dream about. So think good thoughts (Phil. 4:8).

If our mental inputs during the day largely dictate our dream content, then tending to our inputs is a big way we set ourselves up for better dreams. "Our dreams will be apt to follow our foregoing thoughts, and words, and deeds," Richard Baxter observed. "If you think most frequently and affectionately of that which is good, you will dream of that which is good."[12]

In his response to the question about unwanted sexual dreams, Piper wisely suggests purging your movie and TV inputs of all sexually stimulating content. The same principle applies for violent or scary movie and TV content. If at night you're frequently ingesting horror movies—or even just horrifying news headlines—don't be surprised if your dreams are similarly horrifying. Doomscrolling can lead to doomdreaming.

Piper also suggests prayer and Bible reading before bed: "Soak your mind in the Word just before you go to sleep." This is counsel I've given to friends who struggled with demonic dreams: Read the Bible or a devotional, or just listen to Christian music as part of your bedtime routine. Take your anxieties and fears to God in prayer, and allow his peaceful presence to "guard your hearts and your minds in Christ Jesus" (Phil. 4:6–7).

Just as (to quote *Gladiator*) "what we do in life echoes in eternity," what we think about in waking life echoes in our dreams. So orient your thoughts around the things of God. "Take captive every thought to make it obedient to Christ" (2 Cor. 10:5).

John Baíllíe says there is "one way in which we can exercise some control over our dreams, and that is by the proper direction of our thoughts before we retire."[13] Science reinforces this basic spiritual wisdom.

Where our thoughts go when they have free space to wander (not engaging in some specific mental task) is powerfully predictive of where our minds go in dreams. Scientists call it the default mode network (DMN). It's the wandering, daydreaming mode, the mode of our sleep-onset period between lying down and falling asleep. It's a time when the brain tags mental concerns, questions, and incomplete processes "for later processing during sleep." The DMN is so connected to brain activity in REM sleep that some scholars have described the brain state of dreaming as being "enhanced mind wandering."[14]

WAKING OR SLEEPING, THY PRESENCE MY LIGHT

So can you control your dreams? Not fully. Even little children, whose minds usually are not yet tarnished by dark imagery and ideas, struggle with scary dreams. Innocence in waking life is no guarantee of a pristine dream life. Our dreaming consciousness (even from our first years of life) is not untouched by the fall. Yet in the face of the uncontrollability of dreams, we can take consolation in God's ironclad control over all things. In the bad-dream moments in the night, whether you're comforting a crying child or calming yourself down from a jolting nightmare, immediately pray to God. Thank him for his fatherly love and victory over sin and darkness. Meditate on his sovereignty and let it lull you back to sleep. Perhaps the not-real frights in the night can be a training ground for how you respond in prayer and trust when real-life suffering comes your way.

It may be unsettling that you can't really control your dreams. But you can control your waking thoughts, which will inevitably influence your dreams. So set your mind on things above (Col. 3:2).

Contemplate what's true, honorable, just, pure, lovely, commendable, excellent, and praiseworthy (Phil. 4:8). Go to sleep thinking about God's attributes we're pondering in this book: his "never slumbers" sovereignty, his merciful salvation, his abundant grace, his resurrecting power, his ingenious creativity.

Lie down praising your Creator for the miracle of your making and for the awesome possibilities of what *you* can make of the world, both in waking and dreaming life. You are created in the image of a God who dreamed this extraordinary world into existence. Let the words of a beloved Celtic hymn be true of you, your north-star guidance as you think, act, sleep, and dream:

> Be thou my vision, O Lord of my heart;
> Naught be all else to me, save that thou art;
> Thou my best thought, by day or by night;
> Waking or sleeping, thy presence my light.

Pause and Ponder

Pause

Is there a big decision you're contemplating or some area of your life where you are seeking God's guidance? Among other things (such as seeking input from trusted others), consider praying each night before bed that God would give you clarity—confirmation, warning, or some sort of redirection—in your dreams or through someone else's dream. With prudence and wisdom, lean in to the idea that dreams can be a way God directs your path.

Ponder

1. What is your posture toward dreams as vehicles of divine communication? Are you overly open to it—to the point that you read too much into your dreams? Or are you too closed to it—skeptical that God would ever use your dreams that way?
2. What experiences have you had in dreams that felt like spiritual warfare?
3. How do you deal with dreams that leave you feeling dirty or guilty of sin? What are some helpful ways to respond to dreams like this?
4. Have you ever had a dream that altered your life in a specific way? If you're discussing in a group, share these stories with one another.

7

SLEEPING THROUGH STORMS

We're Called to Be a Restful Presence

If you look at the world, you'll be distressed.
If you look within, you'll be depressed.
If you look at God, you'll be at rest.
—Corrie ten Boom

In repentance and rest is your salvation,
in quietness and trust is your strength.
—Isaiah 30:15

Jesus slept. But Scripture references his sleeping explicitly only once.

The scene is famous. Jesus and his disciples are on a boat, crossing to the other side of the Sea of Galilee. A "furious squall" nearly capsizes the boat. Amid the storm, however, "Jesus was in the stern, sleeping on a cushion" (Mark 4:38). His disciples wake him and ask, "Teacher, don't you care if we drown?" Jesus promptly rebukes the wind and tells the waves, "Quiet! Be still!" They obey (v. 39). Jesus then asks his disciples, "Why are you so afraid? Do you still have no faith?" (v. 40). They ask one another, "Who is this? Even the wind and the waves obey him!" (v. 41).

What does it mean that Jesus slept through the storm?

New Testament scholar Benjamin L. Gladd argues that the storm here is not just a scary occurrence in nature but likely a demonic attack meant to thwart Jesus' mission. The setting of the sea is significant, as "God's enemies dwell in the sea," and countless Old Testament texts associate the sea with "death, rebellion, and chaos."[1] The passage immediately precedes the event when Jesus exorcises a legion of demons and casts them into the sea (Mark 5:1–13). And the word *rebuke*, which Jesus uses to calm the storm, is often the word used when Jesus casts out demons (for example, 8:32–33; 9:25).

The implication is powerful. If Jesus can sleep through a violent act of nature, which is also an act of supernatural oppression, there's nothing he can't sleep through. He sleeps in the midst of enemies to an even greater degree than David did (see Pss. 3:5–6; 4:8), but for the same reason: He trusts in God's sovereignty. He sleeps because he knows his Father is awake. He's confident nothing will stop the kingdom's advance.

Jesus models peaceful, trusting sleep. We won't ever have the perfect trust in God he had. But as with everything in our discipleship, we can strive to be more like Christ, emulating his restedness and peace in ways that bear witness to God's sovereignty and draw nervous, sleepless, storm-tossed souls into the stilled waters of God's presence.

FIVE WAYS CHRISTIANS CAN BE A RESTFUL PRESENCE

What does it look like to be a restful presence in today's restless world? How can our habits of sleep and rest be a ministry that serves others? Here are five ways the restful presence of God's people can point others to God's rest.

1. NONANXIOUS PRESENCE

One cause of our age of anxiety is our excessive information awareness brought about by digital technology. Instead of being confronted only with the trials of our immediate lives and local communities, now we daily scroll through an avalanche of the world's crises, calamities, outrages, and traumas. It unsettles and leaves us asking, What can I do about this? Am I doing enough?

We're also anxious because of the comparison pressure served up to us on social media. As we scroll through friends and acquaintances posting #bestlife tableaus, we wonder, Why is my life so boring by comparison? Am I doing enough?

Society is plagued by chronic anxiety in other ways. We've adopted a frenetic pace, oriented supremely on the fleeting now, with little regard for history or the future. This breeds anxiety. Consumer capitalism feeds on and fuels discontentment: You need this product and this experience and this channel and this self-help program in order to be happy. But if discontentment is the seed of consumer capitalism, anxiety is its fruit. And this bad fruit leaves us not nourished but rather feeling spent: financially, emotionally, and spiritually.

In a world like this, where it's easy to lose your nerve and hard to stay calm, Christians can point people to God's rest by exhibiting a nonpanicky, secure, and satisfied rootedness in God.[2]

This restful demeanor must stem from our trust in God, not in our ability to "keep calm and carry on" nor in our aptitude for winning applause or approval. We can rest easy and be calm because our lives are not our own but belong to God.

Being nonanxious doesn't mean being apathetic or disengaged. There are ways anxiety can be good and rightly ordered. Pastor Seth Troutt points to biblical examples of "good anxiety": anxiety out of concern or care for another's welfare, for example (Phil. 2:20; 1 Cor. 12:25), or a pastor's anxiety for his church's health (2 Cor. 11:28).[3] But many contemporary anxieties are *dis*ordered, particularly those arising from doomscrolling. Christians should resist the cultural frenzy of being constantly undone by a barrage of stressful digital information about which we can't take meaningful action.

Instead, our lives should be marked by confidence in God's provision—spiritually and materially—and contentment, whatever the circumstances (Phil. 4:11). As one author states, "Contentment is key to a good night's sleep."[4] Ecclesiastes 5:12 says, "The sleep of a laborer is sweet, whether they eat little or much, but as for the rich, their abundance permits them no sleep." When we're spoiled and entitled, never satisfied and always hungry for more, it's hard to rest. There's more we could be doing and acquiring. Part of our witness in a world of discontentment-driven anxiety is to model the "rare jewel of Christian contentment," which Puritan writer Jeremiah Burroughs says is centered on our satisfaction in God as our "all in all."[5]

In an anxious and discontented world, true, contented rest is found in God alone. Are we modeling this in our lives? Are we inviting others to find it there too?

2. SLUMBER STEWARDED WELL

Prioritizing healthy sleep habits isn't just good for you. It's a way you can love others. The blessings of rest ripple out from us to those in our circles of influence. As a parent, my healthy habits of sleep model something good for my kids, and I might be adding more years to my life with them. By prioritizing rhythms of rest and Sabbath in my household, I'm loving my family by habituating them to healthy patterns I hope they'll carry with them through life.

Sleep-deprived people tend to be grumpy and set an infectiously negative tone. Some of my worst parenting outbursts, scratchiest moments with my wife, and snarkiest comments to coworkers have come on days when I was just too physically tired. Physical fatigue creates mental and emotional fatigue, which leads to short fuses, impatience with others, and a higher propensity to say and do things that hurt others. A sadly common, tragic example of how poor sleep can negatively affect others is drowsy driving, which claims hundreds of lives in car crashes every year. There's a reason we have warning labels not to operate heavy machinery (including cars) while drowsy. Our lack of sleep can kill us over time, or in an instant—and it can kill others.

But good sleep is life-giving to those around us. A well-rested person tends to be a better worker, spouse, parent, and neighbor. Good stewardship of sleep will serve you well in life, but it will also serve those around you, in beautiful ways.

There are also occasions, or extended seasons of life, when your stewardship of sleep looks like sacrificing your ideal so that others can sleep better. Parents do this all the time: forgoing uninterrupted nighttime sleep as they tend to the needs of babies and toddlers; getting up early to make breakfast for the family; staying up late to clean the house from the chaos of the day. As a dad of four I am often exhausted, wishing I could sleep in (even past 7:00 a.m.!) on occasion. But the rarity of luxurious, uninterrupted sleep isn't a source of resentment; it's a reminder that sacrificing so that my family can rest is part of the duty and privilege of fatherhood.

Even if you're not a parent, you likely will have many opportunities to love others by sacrificing your own sleep. Maybe it's staying up late with a friend in a crisis, or not abruptly ending a meaningful conversation or dinner party because it's past your bedtime. Or it could look like choosing to sleep on the creaky sofa so that others get the comfy bed when you're sharing an Airbnb with a group of friends. Perhaps it's a regular practice of getting up before the sun rises in order to methodically work through your prayer list, giving up an hour of sleep to practice intercessory prayer. It might mean keeping watch all night with a sick or dying loved one, sleeping lightly—or not at all—as you listen for their gasps and cries.

There are ways we love others by prioritizing *our* sleeping well, and there are ways we love others by prioritizing *their* sleeping well. In both cases, it's a ministry of spreading rest that glorifies the God of rest.

3. HAVEN OF HOSPITALITY

We live in a disoriented, dislocated, displaced world. Digital technology has rendered us restlessly uprooted and fragmented. We're tired because place and home have receded into the background as the placelessness of online life takes center stage. Other factors—globalization, suburban sprawl, the normalization of frequent geographic moves, remote work giving professionals the chance to do their jobs anywhere—have contributed to this contemporary rootlessness. We're not as embedded in stable places anyway. We're free-agent nomads, restless rolling stones.

Yet even the restless long for the comforts of community and hospitality. That's why your average coffee shop today is full of remote workers locked into screens. These folks have chosen to be tethered to their devices here, in a coffee shop, rather than at home alone. Even in a displaced digital world—or perhaps because of it—we long to be placed in cozy, inviting, communal environments.

This is a vivid way Christians can bear witness to the God of rest. We can create quiet, refreshing, hospitable spaces—in our homes, churches, businesses, classrooms—that function as havens for weary people beleaguered by the tumult and loneliness of contemporary life.

There's a reason accommodations tend to be where travelers spend most of their trip budgets. There's something sacred about where we sleep, relax, and dwell in peace. The hospitality industry demonstrates how powerful an inviting space can be, one that is designed to facilitate good sleep and replenishment for guests.

I've had a few hotel experiences that were especially replenishing. Los Poblanos Inn and Farm in New Mexico, for example (stay here if you're ever in Albuquerque!), or La Loma Jungle Lodge in Panama. Kira and I stayed at this treehouse rainforest hotel, on a chocolate plantation, for three nights over the New Year's holiday early in our marriage. The natural beauty, the open-air rooms with jungle birdsong at dusk and dawn, the communal meals with homemade-chocolate everything, the friendliness of the staff, led by a married couple who built the place. It was sublime. A little picture of heaven.

That's the power of hospitality's invitation: Come and rest here, sleep on this cozy bed we made for you, enjoy this meal we've prepared for you. As we create restful retreats and safe refuges for weary people, we're echoing the invitational heart of our Savior (Matt. 11:28–29), who is preparing a place for us in the new creation (John 14:2–3).

A few years ago, Kira and I gutted a second garage in our house, renovating it into a midcentury-modern guesthouse designed to be comfortable, functional, and beautiful. Over the years it has been a joy to host hundreds of people there: family, neighbors, Airbnb tourists from all over the world, traveling Christian musicians playing concerts in our city, brides on the night before their wedding, even a displaced family who had just lost their home in the 2024 Los Angeles fires. It's a small way we take rest seriously in our home—by inviting others to experience a haven designed to facilitate restful dwelling.

Life is hectic. Look for ways to use what God has given you to invite weary others into an experience of rest. Do you have a vacation home or guest bedroom? Offer it to others as often as you can. Backyard pool? Invite friends over to enjoy a relaxing swim. Open time in your schedule? Offer to babysit an exhausted young couple's kids so they can have a restorative overnight getaway. Business owner or supervisor? Aim for generous vacation-leave policies and do your best to model healthy work-life balance. You're giving your employees the gift of rest by giving them permission to truly be off when they're off the clock.

Through these and many other ways, we can love our neighbor by modeling the heart of our generous, hospitable God.

4. RELATIONAL SAFE PLACE

The isolation of modern life makes us weary. It's a weariness of the technological dynamics of screen-mediated community. (Can I ever really know or be known in a world of carefully constructed avatars?) But it's also a weariness of the existential dynamics of individualism and exhausting self-referentiality.

In his book *The Weariness of the Self*, Alain Ehrenberg argues that the prevalence of depression in contemporary Western cultures has to do with the pressures of individuality and the obligations of self-constructed identity. Far from liberating, "Be who you want to be!" is a burdensome mantra. The autonomous individual charged to seize her own destiny, craft her own personality, and forge her own path ("creating herself by herself") turns out to be "fragile, lacking in being, weary of her sovereignty."[6] The exhausting loneliness of follow-your-heart autonomy makes us miserable. We are social beings, formed by and alongside others. We need others—to share life's burdens and joys with us, to partner with us in striving, and to dwell with us in rest.

This is a powerful way Christians can be a restful presence in a lonely world: through intentional relationships. A good friendship is a refuge of rest in a hectic world. Sometimes you can bear witness to God's rest simply by inviting someone to coffee and sitting with them, listening well, and asking good questions in the hallowed space of unhurried conversation. We draw one another into rest through intentional fellowship: a long meal at a communal table, a group of friends enjoying a drink around a fire pit, a book discussion group, a Bible study, a workout partner, a shared living space. Solitary life in technological bubbles depletes us. We're rejuvenated in the company of others.

It's true that sometimes people need space by themselves. In the Gospels, Jesus often went away by himself, escaping the crowds to pray (for example, in Matt. 14:13; Mark 1:35; Luke 5:16). If you're "peopled out" and need to recharge by yourself for a time, that's great. Sometimes we love people by giving them solitary space to do this. But don't leave people alone for long. Check in regularly. Err on the side of reaching out. People can always say no to your invitation to grab coffee. But in my experience the gesture of asking them is always appreciated. Life is lonely, intense, and depleting. Human connection refills the tank.

Sometimes what is most tiring about contemporary life is that we feel unknown and unseen, fearing there's no one we can be truly honest with or safely confide in. Millions of people are feeling this right now. They live in your neighborhood. They go to your school or church. They work in the cubicle next to you. They're hungry for the rest of a trusted relationship. Consider how you might be this for them.

5. TRUSTWORTHY TRUTH TELLERS

The disconcerting fragility of our post-truth world is a big factor keeping many of us from rest and peace. Online life—where much of what you see and read may be AI generated—has accelerated our collective skepticism. Centuries of secular "progress" have dethroned God as the source of absolutes, replacing him with speak-your-truth subjectivity. But this atomization of truth, into eight billion droplets of ephemeral whims and vibes, leaves the human community fragmented and weary.

Solid truth is a fundamental component of the rest people seek.

We intuitively know that liberating rest will come only when we enter a refuge built on a solid foundation, with sturdy construction and immovable pillars. Until then we'll continue meandering as spiritual refugees in search of shelter. But on which path, to which destination, and for what purpose should we journey? The pilgrims of a post-Christian age need guides who know the way.

This is the most important expression of our calling as ambassadors of the king of rest. We are to call out to wayfaring souls, wherever we encounter them in their wandering, and say, "There is a perfect rest that will answer your restlessness. There is a true north that will give your life direction. Resolution to your longings. Truth that will make it all make sense."

We help people find rest by telling them the truths of Scripture, even the hard truth of repentance. A life of sin and rebellion always leads to restless angst. Only by turning to God in repentance will people find their rest (Isa. 30:15).

Gospel proclamation is the best thing we can do, ultimately, for restless souls. More than anxiety medication, more than a comfortable bed, more than helping them unclutter or reduce hurry in their lives through lifestyle adjustments, they need Jesus himself. "Truly my soul finds rest in God; my salvation comes from him" (Ps. 62:1). Augustine captures it well in what some have called one of the greatest sentences ever written:[7] "You have made us for yourself, and our hearts are restless till they find their rest in thee."

This is the truth that sets us free. This is the truth our restless world needs.

WHAT IS THE WITNESS OF REST?

Above all, the witness of your rest, sleep, and Sabbath points to this: There is a perfectly loving, perfectly sovereign God who perfectly oversees the universe and perfectly secured our salvation through his death and resurrection. True rest comes only as we trust in this God.

Let's be signposts, prophets, and heralds of the gospel of rest. We can cease striving and receive his salvation by grace. We can cast our cares on Christ (1 Peter 5:7). In him we can rest in the storm. He's our ark in the flood (Gen. 7:7), our ram in the thicket (Gen. 22:13), our blood-stained doorpost in the night (Ex. 12:13), our dry ground in the sea (Ex. 14:21–23), our bread in life's hunger (John 6:35), our water in life's thirst (John 4:13–14). This is news a weary world desperately needs.

We are all like wandering sheep (Isa. 53:6), constantly going astray, constantly vulnerable. We wander aimlessly, often directly into danger. Only the Good Shepherd can lead us into a lacking-nothing place: green pastures, still waters, the right paths, refreshment for our souls (Ps. 23:1–3). We rest in peace only as we rest in him.

Our sleep points to him. Our Sabbath points to him. Our rested Christian lives—as nonanxious, good-sleeping, hospitable, relationally inviting, gospel-proclaiming Jesus people—can point to him.

The God of rest, worthy of worship.

Pause and Ponder

Pause

How might you practice hospitality, providing friends, neighbors, and strangers glimpses of God's rest? Take a specific action this week to practice hospitality as an act of facilitating rest for weary people. Maybe you invite someone over for dinner or let a weary mom's kids play in your back yard for a bit so she can have a breather. Maybe you use your home to host a small group or organize a meal train for a family going through a wearying season. Be creative, but specific.

Ponder

1. What are some specific ways you can practice being a nonanxious presence in your family or community?
2. How do your sleep habits affect those around you, either positively or negatively?
3. Think of some of the best hospitality experiences you've ever had, whether sleeping in a hotel or being hosted in someone else's house. What characterizes these experiences, and how did the host (or hotel staff) create a restful environment for you? What can you take from this and apply to your practice of serving others through hospitality?
4. In what sense is gospel proclamation and evangelism a way of spreading rest?

8

HAMMOCKS AND HUMMINGBIRDS

We're Made to Worship God

You will glorify God by resting. One of the highest acts of devotion is to rest in the Lord.
—Charles Spurgeon, "Return unto Thy Rest"

It is good to praise the Lord
    and make music to your name, O Most High,
proclaiming your love in the morning
    and your faithfulness at night,
to the music of the ten-stringed lyre
    and the melody of the harp.
—Psalm 92:1–3

Morning birdsong is one of the most glorious sounds in existence. The dawn chorus, particularly in springtime, reflects creation's instinctual response to sunrise.

Rebirth, renewal, resurrection. The power and glory of God's design.

A song rises in our hearts as we wake, restored by rest and awakened by the sun. It's a song that has played since the dawn of time, when "the morning stars sang together and all the angels shouted for joy" (Job 38:7).

To be awake, alive, in the fullest sense of God's creational intent, is to be a worshiping being. To wake up and want to sing—as the birds do—is as it should be.

> Praise for the singing!
> Praise for the morning!
> Praise for them, springing
> fresh from the Word!

A new day, new wonders to behold, new mercies. New melodies arise. We echo the psalms of morning praise: "Awake, my soul! Awake, harp and lyre! I will awaken the dawn" (Pss. 57:8; 108:2). Singing is a fitting response to another day and another breath. Another reminder that he is risen and death is defeated. God reigns. He is holy, holy, holy.

> Early in the morning
> Our song shall rise to thee.

Music and sunrise go hand in hand.

For more than a decade I've had a playlist titled "Resurrection," which I return to more than any other playlist. It's mostly instrumental—pieces that evoke, often without words, the majesty of resurrection. The playlist includes Copland's "Appalachian Spring," Mahler's "Resurrection Symphony," Wagner's prelude to "Das Rheingold," Max Richter's "On the Nature of Daylight,"

Explosions in the Sky's "First Breath After Coma," and more. As these songs slowly build from quietness to cacophony, they evoke the stirring to life of the waking world—or the rising to new life of the redeemed soul.

Worship is the right response to rest. And rest is a worshipful response to our salvation. Sleeping or waking, resting or working: It's all an opportunity to worship our Creator. It's how he made us. It's why he made us.

Worship is where it all leads.

WORSHIP AS RECEIVING AND RESPONDING

A few times in this book I've talked about inputs and outputs, how so much in God's design seems to reflect this cycle: receiving (input), which, with time, results in giving (output).

Creation everywhere follows this pattern. Our backyard blueberry bushes rehearse it annually: pruned and naked by late summer, then fed by the inputs of sun and water over autumn and winter, finally blossoming in spring little green orbs that eventually become summer blueberries—nourishing, juicy outputs we eat with our morning yogurt or bake into a pie. The cycle repeats, year after year: taking, giving, taking, giving. It's the blueberry plant's song of praise. Living into its created purpose, it glorifies God.

Our worship, too, is an act of receiving and responding. We worship God as we receive him—chiefly the gift of our salvation and union with Christ, who is the yes and amen to all of God's promises, which are ours in him. We worship God as we gladly receive the Spirit's presence and his many gifts. A worshipful life is one of grateful receptivity for what the Father, Son, and Spirit have done for us and in us, for all the triune God has given, gives, and will give.

The graceful abundance of what we receive naturally prompts us to respond—to pour out as we've been poured into, to give because we have received, to work because we have rested, to sing because God has sung over us (Zeph. 3:17). Worship as receiving leads to worship as response. This looks like an angled mirror: We reflect God's glory both horizontally to others and vertically back to him. Our worshipful song echoes outward in the world and upward like the smoke of a burnt offering.

The Christian poet Li-Young Lee talks about how his life and creative work flow from the reality that "it is finished." *"It is finished* makes me cry, *O my God, O my love. Holy, holy, holy,"* Lee says. Indeed, our creative impulse—our praise instinct—is the natural response to living on this side of "it is finished." When we contemplate the momentous inputs of the gospel—our Savior's love for us, our imputed righteousness and eternal inheritance in him—we can't help but pour ourselves out in adoration and praise. As Lee puts it, "All that's left for me is to break the oil over his feet. All that's left are love songs to God."[1]

A worshipful life is like the blueberry plant. Receiving life and bearing fruit. Resting in him and serving his kingdom. Glorifying him through it all.

REST AS WORSHIP: RECEIVE IN TRUSTING GRATITUDE

Rest is an act of worship in both senses. We worship God as we prioritize rest and gratefully receive it. And we worship God as we respond in rest and from rest.

D. A. Carson once said, "Sometimes the godliest thing you

can do in the universe is get a good night's sleep."[2] Godliness correlates with our trust in God's authority. And part of trusting God's authority is receiving rest rather than constantly striving to earn it.

Sleep is a way we physically enact our trust in God's goodness and sufficiency. It's a way we echo the psalmist who wrote, "Return to your rest, my soul, for the LORD has been good to you" (Ps. 116:7). Every time we lay our heads down, we're participating in a liturgy of praise: "I trust you. You are good. My life is not my own. Like the lilies and the sparrows, I belong to you and am sustained by you. You unfailingly provide. Thank you."

Sabbath is a weekly rehearsal of this same idea: trusting God enough to rest, glorifying him as we declare his sufficiency. Sabbath is the church's weekly reminder that rest and worship are beautifully connected. In *Sabbath as Resistance*, Walter Brueggemann calls Sabbath "an acknowledgment that what is needed is given and need not be seized." He contrasts Sabbath with the posture of acquisitiveness, which he calls "the antithesis of thanksgiving, one based in possessions, the other in gifts."[3]

The heart of Sabbath is remembrance and receptivity of God's provision, a conscious letting go of our anxious urge to control, hoard, acquire, nervously scroll or swipe. "Sabbath," Brueggemann writes, helps us recognize that "we live by gift and not by possession, that we are satisfied by relationships of attentive fidelity and not by amassing commodities."[4]

I love his phrase "attentive fidelity." It contrasts with the distracted spirit of half attention that so defines our hyperactive digital age. Central to worship and spiritual formation is relational presence—with God and his people. When we carve out spaces of rest in our lives, we train the muscles of attentive fidelity toward God: his Word, his world, his people, his mission. Just as we love and honor our spouses or our friends by being present with them—giving them our undivided time and attention—so do we love and honor God by pausing our busy lives to contemplate him, seek him in prayer, sing of his greatness, rest in his finished work, and "taste and see" his goodness (Ps. 34:8).

Which leads to the second sense in which rest fuels worship.

REST AS WORSHIP: RESPOND IN ATTENTIVE WONDER

Where we give our time and attention is what our hearts will worship. And in the dizzying digital age, we have ever less time and attention to give. That's why the disciplines of weekly Sabbath, spaces of stillness and rest, and nightly sleep matter spiritually. To grow in our faith, we must grow in our love and worship of God. We need space to do that.

Breathing room to inhale and exhale the aroma of Christ.

But this is harder than ever. As Kelly Kapic observes, "Digital technology allows us to fill every open moment with a quick diversion. . . . Productivity and diversion now rule us, leaving no quiet empty spaces for the mind and body."[5] It's easier than ever to indulge the fleshly tendency to be doing something always, to fill every iota of space in our lives with microbursts of "productivity"—sending another text, aimlessly scrolling social media, checking email. The smartphone sings a siren song of ceaseless temptation, luring us away from every shred of stillness. But this sort of digital multitasking, Brueggeman observes, "yields a divided self, with full attention given to nothing."[6]

Fidgety fingers on phones impede the stillness we need for attentive worship.

Far from its being wasteful, we should see prioritized times of rest, including nightly sleep and weekly Sabbath, as critical to spiritual formation. Even restful leisure holds spiritual value.

Byung-Chul Han says leisure "is not the neighbour of lazy inactivity; it is its opposite. It does not serve the purpose of distraction, but of collecting oneself. Lingering presupposes a gathering of the senses."[7]

Do you have space to linger? Are your times of leisure merely busyness in different forms, or do they help you slow down, think, reflect, and remember God? Do you see rest as merely fuel for optimizing working life, or as spiritually vital acreage for gathering your senses and growing in attentive fidelity and the stirring of your affections toward Christ?

Rest is a gift God gives us so we can better commune with him. When we intentionally receive this gift, we're communicating to him—and to the observing world—that we trust him and desire his presence. We're displaying our priority of praise in a productivity-obsessed world.

Wonder is essential to worship. "If faith is a sanctuary, then our amazement is its outer courts," Martin Schleske writes.[8] But wonder can't be conjured on demand; amazement can't be switched on like a light, two seconds after a TikTok scrolling session and right before you start another load of laundry. Awe requires space. It arises in the processing time between inputs and outputs.

In the quietness and downtime of rest, we can contemplate the wondrous inputs of what God has done. We can piece together thoughts, words, poems of praise, songs of response. We can be still and meditate on the everlasting rest we'll one day have with God and the saints. We can join Richard Baxter in reminding our souls often: "What a sea of love lies before you. Throw yourself in. Swim with the arms of your love in this ocean of his love."[9]

Do we have time in our lives to swim in the sea of God's love? Or are we too busy with the tasks and pleasures of life on the shore?

Byung-Chul Han has a phrase that has stuck with me: "Praise is the Sabbath of language." He's getting at the fact that just as humans find their fullest purpose in the worshipful space of Sabbath, so language finds its fullest expression in the poetics of praise. Indeed, Han believes "the ultimate purpose of language is praise."[10]

Yet often we go through life so frenetically driven by tasks and hurried to-dos that we only ever employ language in a utilitarian way. Whether in hastily typed text messages or AI-assisted rapid-fire emails, we use the fewest words possible to get the point across. But in this rushed mode, language languishes. Part of what we gain in a rested life is a refreshed capacity to use words meaningfully, not as blunt instruments in barbaric hard labor but as harps and lyres that help us find a melody of praise.

Language doesn't reach these heights of praise without first percolating in the inputs of wonder and sensory observation. Our psalms rise not from a vacuum, nor from the three-second results from ChatGPT prompts, but from the rested spaces where our affections are shaped by pondering God and relishing his gifts. Downtime helps us look up. It's amazing how much you can notice with just a few minutes of calm.

God's love and grace are everywhere for us to observe. John Calvin said, "We cannot open our eyes without being compelled to behold him."[11] But in our frenetic scrolling and exhausting schedules, have we crowded out spaces of restful wonder? Are we losing the capacity to behold him because we've already lost the ability to be still?

Slow down. Go sit outside in a hammock, an Adirondack chair in the back yard, a rocking chair on the patio. Go on phone-free walks. Simply observe the beauty and glory around you. Wherever you live, whatever the climate or context, open your eyes. Behold God's glory.

For me it's our backyard avocado tree in March, shedding its old leaves as shimmering neon-green buds of baby fruit begin to form. It's the elegant hummingbirds buzzing around our camellia, searching for pollen and nectar, serving and being served. It's my children hitting baseballs over the roof, giggling on the tree swing, pondering vapor trails in the sky. It's the scent of orange blossoms as white flowers signal future fruit—a citrus perfume that has its moment every spring in SoCal, before the star jasmine becomes the aromatic centerpiece in early summer.

What is it in your part of the world?

Create space to rest so you have time to notice.

TRIGGERS OF HOMEWARD LONGING

The worshipful posture of rest *now* is a foretaste of the unending worship of our eternal Sabbath to come. That holy place of peaceful, praise-filled presence—the seventh-day kingdom for which we were made—beckons to us from eternity's future and Eden's past. Fittingly, it's in spaces of rest where we can hear the call most clearly. Some describe it as *Sehnsucht*. It's a whisper from the wind, a homeward ache in our gut. Now and not yet captured in an inarticulable emotion.

I experience it sometimes when I wake in the morning, satisfied, at peace, cozy in bed, but aware that it's ending. The day's burdens await. I experience it on vacation, when the hectic pace of life feels far away and the splendors of presence abound, yet the awareness of a "back to the grind" ending looms. I experience it at church almost every week, as the fellowship of the worshiping saints teases me with a glimpse of heaven.

When I was a kid, I felt its pang in the last days of summer, when I said goodbye to my cousins after our once a year visit, and when we drove away for the last time from the Redbud Street house of my earliest years. What ties these moments together? It's the bittersweet mixture of satisfied fullness and what G. K. Chesterton coined "divine discontent." It's the grateful acknowledgment that these good things were *so good*. But they are signposts of something better, something beyond this world, yet everywhere advertised. A deeper magic. A purer nourishment. The crystalline headwaters of all goodness, beauty, and truth.

The Source.

What triggers this homeward longing for you? In *This Homeward Ache*, Amy Baik Lee offers a few more examples: "Does music in its most captivating form foreshadow a certain fullness and harmony that our voices will have as we speak with and sing to our Creator? Do we cherish the warm diffused light of the low sideways sun because our souls anticipate the day when the lamp of the New Jerusalem—the Lamb of God, whose glory renders both sun and moon unnecessary (Rev. 21:23)—will dwell with us and beside us?"[12]

Why do certain things in life resonate in the soul, stirring up *Sehnsucht*? Do we delight in afternoon naps in hammocks or a sublime night's sleep because that sense of releasing our grip on life and receiving profound restoration is a foretaste of new-creation life? I don't know. But I suspect God made a lot in this "earthly city" to be pointers toward the City of God to come.

Martin Schleske ponders this about springtime: "Perhaps it is for this reason alone that the earth's axis is tilted and thereby gives us the seasons, so that spring can show our hopelessness that life and beauty can miraculously emerge out of all that seems barren and dead."[13]

Maybe that's also the purpose of sleeping and waking: a daily springtime following the winter of night. Life and beauty emerging from what seems dead. A picture in miniature of God's cosmic redemption.

HYMN OF GRATEFUL PRAISE

Praise him.

Praise him in the morning and the evening. Praise him *for* the morning and the evening. Praise him as you rest and sleep. Praise him *for* the gifts of rest and sleep. Praise him as you work and wake. Praise him *for* the gifts of working and waking life.

> Praise him for his acts of power;
> praise him for his surpassing greatness. . . .
> Let everything that has breath praise the LORD.
>
> —*Psalm 150:2, 6*

Praise him for the sun that governs the day and the moon that governs the night. Praise him for the stars that shimmer like nocturnal diamonds, unfathomably numerous and far from our tiny earthly habitation, yet each one numbered and named (Ps. 147:4).

Praise him for the humming buzz of Los Angeles at rush hour and the great silence of the Mojave Desert at night. Praise him for a just-born baby's amniotic-crusted eyes opening up to the world outside the womb. Praise him for the just-died grandfather whose shriveled hand we've tearfully held as he passed from this world.

Praise him for the heartache and the hope, the perils and the promises, the endings and the beginnings, the toil and the triumph. From the rising of the sun to its going down, praise him (Ps. 113:3).

> For the beauty of each hour
> Of the day and of the night,
> Hill and vale, and tree and flow'r,
> Sun and moon, and stars of light;
> Lord of all, to thee we raise
> This our hymn of grateful praise.

Pause and Ponder

Pause

Write a poem of praise or a letter to God in the style of a biblical psalm. Ideally, do this in some beautiful location where the inputs of God's creation stir your affections to respond to God in the output of poetic praise. If you're a musician, consider turning what you write into a song.

Ponder

1. How do you experience worship as receiving? What about worship as responding? How does this receiving-and-giving dynamic connect to God's design for sleep and rest?
2. What do you think Byung-Chul Han means when he says "praise is the Sabbath of language"?
3. What triggers homeward longing for you? Where do you most feel foretastes of eternity?
4. If it's true that downtime helps us look up, and that a vibrant life of wonder and worship requires us to slow down and notice, what can you do practically to ensure your life has enough downtime?

Part 2

WHAT SLEEP AND REST REVEAL ABOUT GOD

9

ON THE SEVENTH DAY

God Rests

Inactivity has a logic of its own, its own language, temporality, architecture, magnificence—even its own magic.

—Byung-Chul Han, *Vita Contemplativa*

Then God blessed the seventh day and made it holy, because on it he rested from all the work of creating that he had done.

—Genesis 2:3

Stillness makes many of us uncomfortable. To the optimization-minded, the pause of sleep can feel intrusive. We don't like to be forced to stop. Yet God—who certainly had no need to stop—stopped. He had limitless capacity to keep going, doing, and creating, endlessly tinkering like an artist with an infinite canvas and infinite ideas. But he did stop. Genesis 2:2–3 makes this clear by mentioning no less than three times that God did not work on the seventh day.

Clearly this is an important idea. But why? What does it mean that God rested from his work? God doesn't sleep or grow weary (Isa. 40:28). He doesn't need anything, including rest. And yet Genesis 2 is clear. God chooses rest. How are we to understand the meaning of this divine seventh-day rest?

We can't think of God's rest as a powering down prompted by exhaustion. Nor can we think of it as an anticlimactic coda after the rollicking symphony of a six-day explosion of creativity. If anything God's rest on the seventh day is the climax of the creation sequence described in Genesis 1, not an afterthought.

The first five days of creation God sees as good.

The sixth day's creation of Adam and Eve he sees as very good.

The seventh day he blesses and makes holy.

The sequence goes from good to very good to holy. Here at the beginning of Scripture, at the beginning of human history, God elevates rest to the highest place, and this elevation persists as the biblical narrative progresses. He creates the day of rest for all humans "in order to point to the goal of human existence, namely, eschatological life with God."[1]

This hallowed seventh-day rest is not a postscript ending as much as a true commencement. Construction is complete, and creation can now be enjoyed in the presence of the Creator. Communion can commence. And even though it marks the seventh of seven days in a sequence, God's rest here is more a beginning than an ending. It's a thesis statement that sheds light on everything that follows in redemptive history.

On this first seventh day, God is enthroned and present with God's people in God's place. Eden is a place of perfect *shalom*—peace. All is well.

Paradise is lost after the fall, however. The God-people-place harmony is broken. When Adam and Eve are banished from the garden (Gen. 3:23–24), human access to God's rest is revoked.

Yet the story of Scripture is one of a gracious God pursuing his people by providing progressively richer foretastes and glimpses of his divine rest: deliverance from Egyptian captivity, the institution of the Sabbath, taking up residence in the promised land, and ultimately the victory of Jesus Christ, the Lord of the Sabbath, who is the solution for our restlessness and secures an eternal Sabbath rest for the people of God (Heb. 4:1–11).

On this first seventh day, God's rest is the pinnacle of perfection: peace, security, beauty, joy. And in the "seventh day" of eternity described in the Bible's closing book, God's rest is once again the pinnacle of perfection: no more tears, pain, death, sadness; only communion with the creator God, who, as ever, is making all things new (Rev. 21:5).

God, once again and forevermore, will be enthroned and present with God's people in God's place. Eden is restored. A seventh-day rest that will never end, for all who are in him.

REST AS HOLY TIME

Redemptive history is, in many ways, a history of God's rest and our relationship to it. In the fall, we lost access to God's rest. And in the gospel, we gain eternal access to God's rest.

In *The Holiness of God*, R. C. Sproul says, "The whole scope of redemptive history, from start to finish, is made sacred in the observance of the Sabbath,"[2] which points us back to God's work of creation and redemption and forward to the inheritance achieved by that redemption: our future Sabbath rest in heaven. Another biblical scholar calls Sabbath "a microcosm of human history—creation, redemption, and consummation."[3] Every Sabbath in this life is a temporal glimpse of the permanent, eternal rest to come.

When God blessed the seventh day and made it holy, he introduced a sort of sacred time set apart from all other time. Abraham Heschel points out that nothing else in the creation account—no object or space—was deemed holy in the first chapter of Genesis. Only time was hallowed, the seventh day: "When history began, there was only one holiness in the world, holiness in time."[4]

Heschel describes our keeping the Sabbath day as "a paraphrase of His sanctification of the seventh day."[5] Our observance of a holy Sabbath day is only the faintest glimpse of God's holy rest, but it is still potent. It regularly reorients our lives around God and eternity, breaking the hold of temporal, passing things and stirring our hearts to long for home in him.

I think about the deep peace and rest I feel sitting on the sand watching the ocean waves near our home in Southern California. The comforting rhythms of unending waves—coming from an unfathomably vast, powerful ocean—provide me with a sublime assurance that one day I'll be on heaven's bright shore, enjoying the awesome power and ceaseless love of God up close, forever: wave after wave after wave—times infinity. I think about those Sundays of my childhood when, after singing "Wonderful Grace of Jesus" (or other classics from our Baptist hymnal), we'd enjoy a postchurch potluck in the fellowship hall. In spite of imperfect singing and very imperfect casseroles, these moments unmistakably pointed me to the perfect to come.

So it goes with the holy moments in life, both on Sabbath and in every little gift of bountiful rest and precious peace, including a good sleep. These are echoes and paraphrases of the rest our restless souls so deeply desire.

To enter God's rest is to enter the hallowed seventh-day place of security under God's perfect rule; it is to be free of all that makes us rest-less. And what is it that makes us most restless? Our sin. Think of Adam and Eve in Eden. They had everything, including access to God's rest. But their sin made them squirmy: ungrateful, untrusting, unsatisfied with God's rule in God's perfect place. They wanted more.

Sin is placing ourselves on the throne, assuming we can rule our lives better than God can. This is not only deadly, it's exhausting. By contrast, living joyfully under God's rule—being content with him on the throne—is where we find life and rest.

Rest is holy, ordered, and content in stark contrast to restlessness, which is often a product of unholiness, disorder, and discontentment. To trust God with all our hearts rather than leaning on our own understanding makes it easier to be both holy and rested. If we truly believe God is on the throne, sovereign and in control, having "overcome the world" (John 16:33) in spite of persisting troubles, we can rest easier.

Entering God's perfect rest always goes hand in hand with acknowledging his perfect rule.

REST AS JOYFUL, GRATEFUL ATTENTIVENESS

Rest is more like an exclamation point than an asterisk. Again, the day of rest is the only one of the seven that God makes holy. Rest is set-apart space for worship. And worship is the point.

As we've seen already in this book, sleep and rest can be times of heightened awareness and focused attention when our perception is clearer and our humanity is optimized. That sounds counterintuitive. We're most optimally human at rest? Even when we're asleep? Yes. This is one of the surprising dynamics of God's economy of grace. If all we ever do is produce, we can never partake. If our lives are ceaseless striving for mere survival, our humanity atrophies, and we miss opportunities to glorify God and enjoy him.

WHAT SLEEP AND REST REVEAL ABOUT GOD

Animals survive. Humans enjoy. It's a crucial part of what defines us as image-bearing beings.

To be sure, we glorify God by working too. Producing, creating, and ordering chaos is worship. But there's a special genre of worship that's possible in the "pause" space of rest. Tim Keller says of the seventh day, "God did not just cease from his labor; he stopped and enjoyed what he had made."[6] Judith Shulevitz, in her excellent book *The Sabbath World*, says, "God stopped to show us that what we create becomes meaningful only once we stop creating it and start remembering why it was worth creating in the first place. . . . We have to remember to stop because we have to stop to remember."[7]

Obviously God is not forgetful. He didn't need to stop in order to remember, but he chose to stop as a way to help us remember. By pausing to honor the just-created creation, God forever dignifies the act of taking time to enjoy beauty and praise the maker of that beauty. Any artist (or really anyone who has created some labor of love) can attest to the importance of having a moment to celebrate and enjoy the creation: the gallery opening of an artist's new show, the red carpet premiere of a filmmaker's movie, the ribbon cutting ceremony of a newly constructed building. These festive moments are hallowed in their own way, and they demonstrate the idea that rest for us is not only a needed break from hard work, it's often the culmination and festive commemoration of it.

If we could bottle the seventh-day feeling, it would be akin to the experience of communing after creating, celebrating after striving, praising after preparation. It's like the moment of sitting down at a perfectly set table and saying a prayer of gratitude before enjoying an extravagant feast, following hours of laborious kitchen prep. It's the bliss a newly married couple experiences on the honeymoon after months of engagement, wedding planning, and all the work that preceded their union. John Walton compares the seventh-day feeling to the experience of finally being settled in a home after unpacking boxes, putting up drapes, and going through the setup activities after moving into a new house. The seventh day is when the house became home.[8]

God's rest is like all of these blissful feelings, but infinitely more sublime and for all eternity.

REST AS ENGAGED PRESENCE, NOT CHECKED-OUT ABSENCE

God's rest gives an impression not of disengaged zoning out but of heightened senses. Sabbath's holy time is an affirmation rather than a negation. Genesis 2:2 uses the Hebrew word *sabat*, from which *sabbath* is derived, and it has the basic meaning of "ceasing." But it's a ceasing that leads not to nothingness but to a positive state of safety, security, and stability. It is not rest *from* but rest *in*. God "does not require rest *from* either cosmic forces or human disturbances but seeks rest *in* a dwelling place,"[9] a dwelling place that in Psalm 132 (vv. 7–8, 13–14) is repeatedly equated with a resting place. Psalm 132 "pulls together the ideas of divine rest, temple and enthronement," Walton observes. "After creation, God takes up his rest and rules from his residence."[10]

Divine rest isn't divine disengagement. It is God assuming his place on the throne and commencing his rule—in his place, with his people. And it is because this king is ruling that this kingdom is a restful place. Here's how Walton sums it up: "Resting pertains to the security and stability found in the equilibrium of an ordered system. When God rests on the seventh day, he is taking up his residence in the ordered system that he has brought about in the previous six days. It is not something that he does only on the seventh day; it is what he does every day thereafter."[11]

God's rest is the outcome of his perfect rule and perfect

holiness. It overflows to all those who put their trust in his rule. Our stillness is tied to our recognition of his authority (for example, Ps. 46:10). And our inability to trust him keeps us from entering his rest (for example, Heb. 3:11; Ps. 95:11).

We achieve rest insofar as we know in our gut that God has already achieved rest for us.

GOD OF GRACIOUS GRATUITY, NOT MERCILESS UTILITY

Have you ever thought about where our seven-day week comes from, with one of the days set aside for nonworking time? It's here. Genesis 2.

Dividing time into seven-day periods—including one day to rest—was not a normal practice in the ancient Near East.[12] When Maggie Smith's aristocratic countess on *Downton Abbey* uttered her classic line, "What is a weekend?" she could have been speaking for all people in ancient history. The world has Judaism to thank for introducing the novel—and glorious!—idea of a regular day of rest.

What kind of God would structure time this way? What kind of God would institute a day of holy rest? He didn't need to do it. He's never tired and needs no reprieve from work. But that's the point. God's rest isn't about utilitarian need; it's about gratuitous love. It's significant that a day of rest is the first thing Adam and Eve experience after they are made on day six. Humans awaken to existence, and their first full day they spend living at rest, not at work. What a gift. What grace.

God is perfectly at rest in himself. He needs no object of love beyond himself. Yet as an utterly free act, he created us for his glory, and we glorify him by entering his rest.

God's seventh-day pattern of rest is a gift for our good. He prioritizes it—even calls it holy—so his followers will prioritize it too, like "a father setting an example for his children."[13] He does this because he loves us. Because he's a God of superabundant grace.

We'll explore this aspect of God more in chapter 12. For now we'll end this chapter by marveling at the fact that God's gratuitous love was present right at the world's creation. His seventh-day rest reveals who he is and how he wants us, the crown of his creation, to live.

In a merciless, cutthroat, always-on world, God wants his people to experience rest. We can take a day off without stressing, knowing the world is in good hands with God on the throne.

Pause and Ponder

Pause

Carve out a few minutes of your day to be silent and undistracted. Seek God in prayer, praising him, thanking him for his secure peace and rest. Read Psalm 16, 23, 132, or one of your favorite psalms. Let this quiet time with the God of rest be a foretaste of the perfect rest to come.

Ponder

1. Ponder the idea of "holiness in time." What does it look like to encounter God's holiness not in space but in time?
2. Does anything in this chapter make you think

differently about what you imagine it will be like to enter God's divine rest in eternity?

3. What does Sabbath rest have to do with the gospel?

10

CREATION WORKS AND SLUMBERS

God Is an Intentional Designer

Polarity, or action and reaction, we meet in every part of nature; in darkness and light; in heat and cold; in the ebb and flow of waters; in male and female; in the inspiration and expiration of plants and animals. . . . An inevitable dualism bisects nature, so that each thing is a half, and suggests another thing to make it whole.

—Ralph Waldo Emerson, "Compensation"

God called the light "day," and the darkness he called "night." And there was evening, and there was morning—the first day.

—Genesis 1:5

In the previous chapter we took a deep-dive look at God's seventh-day rest. But what God made in the first six days of creation also reflects his value of rest. His design for creation is unmistakably marked by a rhythmic complementarity between work and rest, activity and stillness, waking and sleeping, day and night.

From top to bottom, in all its vastness, God's creation is colored by complementary motifs. All creatures have periods of rest (if not legitimate sleep) coupled with periods of activity. What this looks like varies across species, often in fascinating ways. For example, marine mammals sleep, but they do so while still swimming! How this works is a brilliant evidence of an ingenious creator. Research on dolphins and whales has shown that they have unihemispheric sleep, meaning one half of their brains sleeps while the other half stays awake to survive through necessarily ceaseless movement in the ocean. This split-brain sleeping also occurs in birds, allowing them to keep one eye open for environmental threats while the other eye can sleep.[1]

The complementary motif of rest/activity is also evident in plant life, with almost all known plants exhibiting cycles of dormancy (rest) and activity (growth and fruitfulness). The seasons reflect it too. Based on the tilt of the earth's axis relative to its position around the sun, there are some seasons of fruitfulness (spring and summer) and some for fallow rest (winter). In a way, every twenty-four-hour day reflects it in microcosm: At dawn we wake from slumber, like the first tulips or daffodils rising from bulbs in the ground (spring). Soon our activity/fruitfulness reaches its prime, around midmorning or midday (summer), after which we start to grow tired again, as the day progresses (fall). And as the sun sets and darkness encroaches, we prepare for and ultimately settle into sleep/dormancy (winter).

When you start to look for it, you notice rest-activity duality everywhere. The ocean tides are an ebb and flow of activity and passivity. Volcanoes go through cycles of activity and dormancy. So do black holes. Sleep and wake, rest and activity: It's a harmonious, ordering logic that pervades God's creation.

This logic was there from the beginning, even before the fall. Adam was sleeping before the fall (Gen. 2:21). Sleep wasn't a result of the fall (though certainly our trouble sleeping and the many types of sleep disorders are). It's not just a necessary evil. Dormant periods and long stretches of seeming barrenness—when the landscapes seem brown and the trees naked—aren't a mistake of creation. They're purposeful.

Rest was there at the beginning, and so was work: not punishments destined ever to be at odds but gifts ever to be in life-giving balance.

REST AND WORK AS COMPLEMENTARY PAIR

God created the world in complementary polarities:

- Light and darkness (Gen. 1:4)
- Day and night (Gen. 1:5)
- Waters above and waters below (Gen. 1:6–8)
- Land and seas (Gen. 1:9–10)
- Sun and moon (Gen. 1:14–18)
- Male and female (Gen. 1:27)
- Work and rest (Gen. 1:28; 2:2–3)

The pairing of sleep and wakefulness is not explicitly mentioned in the Genesis creation account, but presumably it was a natural byproduct of things that are mentioned (light/dark, day/night, sun/moon). So from the beginning, the coupling of sleep and wakefulness existed alongside an entire creation imbued by God with the logic and beauty of complementarity. And even after he destroyed creation with the flood because of human wickedness,

God's postflood promises to Noah include this reassertion of nature's complementary balance:

> As long as the earth endures,
> seedtime and harvest,
> cold and heat,
> summer and winter,
> day and night
> will never cease.
>
> —*Genesis 8:22*

We should note a few things about these creational polarities. First, they aren't perfectly symmetrical. For example, there are only two days in the year (the spring and fall equinox) when every part of earth experiences roughly equal amounts of day and night. The vast majority of time, the temporal relationship between day and night is asymmetrical and ever changing. The same is true of summer and winter's duration, or land and sea's size. The planet isn't a fifty-fifty split of oceans and dry ground. It's 30 percent land and 70 percent sea. And consider the rhythm of work and rest God designed and modeled: not half work and half rest but six days of work and one day of rest. Likewise, some of us might wish we could spend half of our day sleeping. But the average person gets closer to seven hours of sleep per night, leaving seventeen hours of each day for waking activity. This balance—with more weight given to work than rest—is by God's design.

Things can be complementary, balanced, equally valuable, and harmonious without being absolutely symmetrical. This is one mind-blowing aspect of God's creation: It's all so finely tuned for life and flourishing, but in unexpected ratios and asymmetry.

A second observation about the complementary couplings in God's creation: They are not oppositional categories or dueling sides in a battle for supremacy. It's not as if the sun and moon are competing for a privileged place. Rather, each has its own time and purpose, taking shifts governing day or night. They work together in harmony. Sometimes these complementary relationships look like constant give and take, as in the land and sea with their endless dance of tidal patterns, erosion, and ever-changing coastlines. But it's a mutually beneficial give-and-take, designed by a loving God. Think of the hydraulic cycle. The clouds give water as precipitation but then take it back again via evaporation. Down and up, give and take, repeated every day around the world. They are two essential sides of the same organic cycle, created to sustain life on earth. One without the other wouldn't work. Far from competitors, they collaborate in a coherent way we marvel to behold.

The same is true of the pairings we're focused on in this book: work and rest, waking and sleeping. Work is a great blessing, as is being awake and alert, able to perceive and contribute to the world. But would work be a blessing without rest? Would waking life be a blessing without sleep? No. To work ceaselessly with no break or to be awake constantly with no ability to sleep would be hellish. Maybe hell will be the opposite of eternal rest, a constant state of forced labor, exhaustion, and restlessness.

There's a scary (and thankfully rare) genetic sleep disorder called fatal familial insomnia (FFI). Those with this terrible disease struggle to sleep and eventually become essentially unable to sleep. FFI unfolds like a living nightmare—first panic attacks, hallucinations, and worsening insomnia, followed by decline in cognitive function, dementia, rapid weight loss, difficulty breathing and walking, muscle atrophy, and finally a coma from which you never wake up. From the onset of symptoms, the average FFI patient dies within eighteen months. There is no cure.

What does permanent wakefulness do to you? It eventually kills you. One well-publicized victim of FFI is Chicago music teacher Michael Corke, who in 1993 died at the age of forty-two, having not slept for six months.[2] We can't survive without sleep.

Yet *only* sleeping would be a sort of death too. People who struggle with mental illness often find it difficult to get out of bed; waking life is too much to bear. "Bed rotting" is an emerging term for a stress and anxiety coping mechanism where people spend all day in bed as a form of self-care. But bed rotting and sleeping too much can result in bedsores, muscle atrophy, and a litany of other health risks associated with a sedentary lifestyle. As an escape from the challenges of life, bed rotting becomes a form of death. Those who are alive but in a coma or prolonged sedation also capture the not-ideal nature of an always-sleeping state. We weren't created for constant sleep.

Wakefulness and sleep are good things only in relationship with one another. The same is true of work and rest.

The show *Severance* demonstrates this vividly. By portraying characters who have severed the healthy pairing of work and rest and compartmentalized them as separate conscious experiences, the show makes clear that a life of only work or only rest would be miserable.[3] The latter point is prophetic in our technological moment, as AI experts predict that in a matter of years, human work will be done mostly by robots and jobs will no longer be necessary. It may sound like utopia to some, but in reality that potential future would be dystopian. We are created to work. We are created to rest. Not one or the other. Both.

God built the rhythmic pairing of work and rest into creation for a reason. Things go awry when God's creation, whether humans or animals or even the land itself, is only resting but never working, or only working and never resting. Some animals need to hibernate. But if they only hibernated and never hunted or gathered food, they would die. The land needs rest from productivity. Scripture even gives us imagery of the land "enjoying" its rest (Isa.

14:7; 2 Chron. 36:21; Lev. 26:34). But the land was also created to produce.

Productivity is a good thing. But never-ending productivity is counterproductive in both the land and us. We heal, we replenish, and we are fruitful not just because we rest and sleep but, as we have seen, *while* we rest and sleep. This is the miraculous order of things in God's universe.

When we trust this good design, we flourish. When we reject it or doubt it, thinking rest is a waste of time and sleep is for losers, we go against the grain of God's order and do ourselves harm. Trust God's wisdom as a designer! The ordered polarities he created aren't meant to give us whiplash. They're meant to keep us steady.

WHICH IS THE HIGHER STATE?

Humans aren't great at recognizing the both-and benefits of complementary things. We feel more comfortable with hierarchies, such that even if we see some value in two parts of a pairing, we still elevate one over the other.

This has been true of sleep/rest and wakefulness/work. Aristotle, for example, argued that while sleep "belongs of necessity to each animal," the waking state is "its highest end."[4] Probably most people throughout history have agreed with this. Sleep is necessary, but waking life is superior.

Others argue the opposite. Prominent sleep scientist Matthew Walker goes so far as to ask, "What if sleep is so useful—so physiologically beneficial to every aspect of our being—that the real question is: Why did life ever bother to wake up? Considering how biologically damaging the state of wakefulness can often be, that is the true evolutionary puzzle here, not sleep."[5]

Abraham Heschel argues, "The Sabbath is not for the sake of the weekdays; the weekdays are for the sake of the Sabbath. It is not an interlude but the climax of living."[6] Byung-Chul Han says "inactivity constitutes the human" and "the ultimate purpose of all human endeavor is inactivity."[7] Josef Pieper claims, "Leisure does not exist for the sake of work—however much strength it may give a man to work; the point of leisure is not to be a restorative, a pick-me-up, whether mental or physical; and though it gives new strength, mentally and physically, and spiritually too, that is not the point. Leisure, like contemplation, is of a higher order than the *vita activa*."[8]

Some Christians and Jews point to the phrase repeated throughout Genesis 1, "And there was evening and there was morning," to signal the completion of a day's work. This is why in Jewish tradition, the day begins not with dawn but with sunset: evening first, then morning. In *Liturgy of the Ordinary*, Tish Harrison Warren ponders how "powerfully reorienting, even jarring," this understanding of time is for those of us inclined to measure days by our own accomplishments: "The Jewish day begins in seemingly accomplishing nothing at all. We begin by resting, drooling on our pillow, dropping off into helplessness."[9]

Eugene Peterson says this evening-morning sequence "conditions us to the rhythms of grace": "We go to sleep, and God begins his work. As we sleep he develops his covenant. We wake and are called out to participate in God's creative action. We respond in faith, in word. But always grace is previous. Grace is primary. We wake into a world we didn't make, into a salvation we didn't earn. Evening: God begins, without our help, his creative day. Morning: God calls us to enjoy and share and develop the work he initiated."[10]

It's interesting to think about two very consequential moments of human sleep in the biblical narrative, both of which use the same Hebrew word, *tardema* ("deep sleep"): Adam's deep sleep (Gen.

2:21) and Abram's deep sleep (Gen. 15:12). In both cases, a moment of apparent human inactivity is the occasion for a moment of profound productivity on God's part. While Adam slept, God created Eve for him, making possible the covenantal union of marriage and the fruitfulness of offspring. While Abram slept, God established his covenantal union with him and reinforced his promise of many offspring. In both cases it was God who took the initiative and did the work and man who received the grace. Both men went on to be fruitful, but it's a fruitfulness made possible by God's prior grace, received as they slept. These deep-sleep moments powerfully juxtapose Adam's and Abram's passivity with God's activity, removing any inkling that we achieve greatness from the launchpad of our own talents. No, we are fruitful *from* God's gifts. Our productivity follows—flows from—God's.

We rest and then work.
We were dead and then alive.
We give because we first received.
We love because he first loved us (1 John 4:19).
And there was evening, and there was morning.

ETERNAL HARMONY OF GIVING AND RECEIVING

To emphasize the importance of this order (evening first, then morning; rest before work) is not to imply a hierarchy, however. It remains true that evening and morning, rest and work, sleeping and waking, have no meaning apart from the other. We sometimes sleep because we are sometimes awake, and vice versa.

Fourth-century church father Gregory of Nyssa describes the relationship between sleep and waking in this way: "Neither of these abides continually, but both give way, each at the other's coming; nature thus by their interchange so renewing herself."[11] It's a beautiful way of capturing God's ingenious design in seamlessly weaving together these polarities, "each at the other's coming," such that renewal—life—is the result.

The language of giving and receiving captures it well. In waking life we give, make contributions, pour ourselves out. In sleep we receive, accept deposits, fill up anew. The day gives illumination, warmth, and conditions for activity. At night we receive sensory relief, cooler temperatures, and conditions for rest. The land and sea are constantly trading sediment and particles of life. The waters above and the waters below are likewise in a daily dance of give and take.

So much in creation follows this general pattern. Why? Perhaps it's because the God who created this universe is himself the perfection of this pattern.

Within what Fred Sanders calls "the happy land of the Trinity," there is an eternally existing tripersonal love characterized by the unending "love of the Father for the Son, and the Son for the Father, in the unity of the Holy Spirit."[12]

Consider what God the Son says in his inter-Trinitarian prayer to God the Father in John 17:5: "And now, Father, glorify me in your presence with the glory I had with you before the world began." What was this glory the Trinity had before the world existed? It was the glory of endlessly giving and receiving love, honor, and praise in perfect fellowship. D. A. Carson says John 17:5 is "a picture of God whose love, even in eternity past, even before the creation of anything, is other-oriented. . . . There has *always* been an other-orientation to the love of God. All the manifestations of the love of God emerge out of this deeper, more fundamental reality: love is bound up in the very nature of God. God is love."[13]

We also see the dynamic in how the Trinity's tripersonal love within itself overflows to us via the Son's gracious love: "As the

Father has loved me, so have I loved you" (John 15:9). Carson says that in this verse "we move from the intra-Trinitarian love of the Father for the Son, to the Son's love of his people in redemption. . . . Receiving love, so has he loved."[14]

God wants us to do the same. Having first received love, we respond—by the power of the Holy Spirit—in love: first to God with all our hearts, souls, and minds, and then to our neighbor (Matt. 22:37–39). God's love precedes everything. It makes all subsequent love possible. As John famously writes, "This is love: not that we loved God, but that he loved us and sent his Son as an atoning sacrifice for our sins. Dear friends, since God so loved us, we also ought to love one another" (1 John 4:10–11).

We get the clearest picture of the glorious love of God in this gospel, in the special revelation of God's Word. But God's world reinforces it, even if the pictures are less clear. In its many varieties of complementary relationships—day and night, waking and sleeping, work and rest, land and sea, male and female—creation bears witness to a creator whose other-oriented love isn't frozen in place but is always gushing forth in mysterious dynamism, giving and receiving so constantly that the line between the two sometimes blurs.

Maybe the deepest theological resonance in the polarities and contrasts of creation is not in their differences and alternating rhythms but rather in the moments and places where they come together as one. Maybe this is why sunsets and sunrises strike our hearts as the most beautiful times of day: the oneness where day and night merge. Maybe it's why coastlines—where land and sea fuse into a fluid, pulsating blend—are the places humans most desire to visit and live. Maybe it's why the one-flesh union of male and female in marriage is described in Scripture as a mysterious picture of the gospel (Eph. 5:31–32).

Maybe it's like those moments in our work when we get into

such flow that it feels utterly pleasurable, like leisure. Work and rest blend. Maybe it's like that thin-place moment on a Friday late afternoon, when work starts tapering off into rest, or the work we do is merely to set the table for a feast or prepare the house for the weekend.

It's that ephemeral dusk invocation when the sun drops and the moon rises, when the sky is purple and the Sabbath candles are lit, when all seems in balance and the actions of receiving and giving feel like one thing.

Maybe this is what entering God's eternal rest will feel like—the Sabbath-inaugurating sunset feeling, forever.

Pause and Ponder

Pause

This chapter mentions a number of ways God's complementary motif of rest/activity shows up throughout his creation. Where else do you see it? Go outside on a walk, maybe visit a park or some green space, and spend time observing God's handiwork. Where do you see this signature of the Creator—complementary polarities—on display?

Ponder

1. What do you think about the claim that wakefulness and sleep, as well as work and rest, are good things only in relationship with one another? Where have you seen the imbalance of these create problems?

2. This chapter explores the duality of rest and activity as "a harmonious, ordering logic that pervades God's creation." What does this look like in your life or your family's life? Do your rhythms of rest and activity feel proportionate and harmonious, or out of balance and chaotic?
3. Why do you think what we call beauty so often involves the times or places when two opposites come together—whether the night-day meeting at sunset, the land-sea meeting on a shoreline, or a man-woman meeting in a romance? How does this reflect the imprint of God, who is the author and embodiment of beauty?

11

REMEMBER THE SABBATH

God Creates a Distinct People Through Rest

The Sabbath, said the rabbis, is a bride given by God to her groom, the people of Israel. Once a week, they go forth in wedding clothes to marry her.
—Judith Shulevitz, *The Sabbath World*

Say to the Israelites, "You must observe my Sabbaths. This will be a sign between me and you for the generations to come, so you may know that I am the Lord, who makes you holy."
—Exodus 31:13

Sabbath is a sign (Ex. 31:13; Ezek. 20:12). It points to bigger truths. The practice marks off God's people in multiple ways, communicating distinct truths about the God we worship and the nature of our salvation in him. What are those truths?

In this chapter we'll ponder seven senses in which Sabbath is a sign. Each of these motifs connects to the broader creational categories of rest and sleep, as we've seen and will continue to see in this book. The God who created Sabbath, after all, is the same God who created sleep. Sabbath is liturgical rest, and sleep is biological rest. Both teach theological lessons with plenty of overlap.

Sabbath is a big topic. Countless books have been devoted to it. What follows is only a cursory glance at a few layers of a biblical idea that is foundational for any theological analysis of rest and sleep.

1. SABBATH IS IMITATION

When God gives the fourth commandment at Sinai ("Remember the Sabbath day by keeping it holy," Ex. 20:8), he codifies the pattern he established in the beginning (Gen. 2:2–3), explicitly tying the pattern of six-days labor, seventh-day rest to his example (Ex. 31:17).

One of the foundational ways Sabbath is a sign, then, is that our own pattern of working and resting points to God's. We imitate God, however imperfectly, by working and resting. As Herman Bavinck says, "As it does for God himself, man's work ends in resting, enjoyment, pleasure."[1]

The Sabbath is not holy because we practice it perfectly. Sabbath's holiness does not originate with us. The holiness rather radiates from the perfection of God, whom we faintly picture as we diligently work and intentionally rest. God intends Sabbath to be a practical, rhythmic tether that connects him to his people, a synchronized rhythm that shows the world we are his and he is ours. As we imitate God by keeping the Sabbath, we worship him in the manner of an angled mirror: We reflect his glory both upward to him and outward to the world.

2. SABBATH IS SEPARATION

Sabbath also separates us from worldly values: ceaseless striving, self-reliance, idolatry, insatiable consumerism, hustle-and-grind pace. Countercultural separation is part of the nature of Sabbath (or in Hebrew *Shabbat*).

In her book *The Sabbath World*, Judith Shulevitz describes how Jews mark the end of Shabbat with a ritual called Separation (Havdalah) on Saturday night, which includes the saying of blessings like, "Blessed are you, God, because you separate the holy from the everyday, the light from the darkness, the people of Israel from everyone else, the seventh day from the six days of creation."[2]

The set-apartness of the Sabbath is a profound source of its power. It's so different from the other six days. Instead of working to achieve, we rest and enjoy. Instead of competing, we commune. Instead of giving, we receive. Instead of keeping to a frantic schedule and constantly checking our phones, Sabbath releases us to be still, offline, at peace. I love how Abraham Heschel describes it: "In the tempestuous ocean of time and toil there are islands of stillness where man may enter a harbor and reclaim his dignity. The island is the seventh day."[3]

If this sounds refreshing, but a bit unrealistic, consider what you might do to practice the separateness of Sabbath. Maybe it starts with simple tweaks like no social media for a day. If you're tempted to work on Sabbath, try putting do-not-disturbs on your devices for the day. Consider going outside—for a walk, a hike, a nap in the hammock—instead of scrolling on screens. "The Sabbath prefers natural light to artificial lights," A. J. Swoboda writes in *Subversive Sabbath*. "The Sabbath returns us to natural light—to the established rhythms of God—and honors sunlight over iPhone light."[4]

Lean in to the countercultural separation of Sabbath. This is a potent way your practice is a sign—perhaps even an invitation—to a weary world desperate for relief.

3. SABBATH IS COMMUNION

Sabbath isn't solitary. It's about communion, both with God and with others. In a world whizzing by in jarring noise and frenetic distraction, Sabbath is about presence, temporally and relationally. Eugene Peterson describes it as "keeping company with God in the present, in the now: attending, adoring."[5] We also keep company with the saints. Sabbath is a "day of sacred assembly" (Lev. 23:3), not a habit of solo piety.

This contrasts with the "iWorld" of contemporary digital culture: chiefly oriented around personal convenience and individual preference. In today's world, even in Christian circles, #sabbathing has become a popular practice for individuals as part of their personal spiritual disciplines. But when our sabbathing practices are solitary ventures—say, taking some time to pray and journal on the beach or in a cabin in the woods—they defeat the purpose of the sacred assembly. They start to look more like secular wellness hacks than sacred worship.

Sabbath is not just for you, an individual. It's for you, plural: the people of God. It's a coming together, not an experience in isolation. Heschel echoes Jewish tradition when he describes Sabbath as a bride and the celebration of Sabbath as "like a wedding."[6] This is a day for covenant renewal between God and his people. Invite guests. Pop open bubbly. Toast. Lock arms. Sing. Dance.

The relational dimension of Sabbath is critical. This is why the Jewish practice of Shabbat involves family meals (often with guests) and gatherings at synagogues. It's why the Christian practice of

Sabbath involves congregational worship at church, the communal ordinance of the Lord's Supper, and sometimes a nicer than normal family meal after church. These festive, worshipful gatherings are meant to be weekly previews of the wedding feast to come.

Don't minimize the relational aspects of Sabbath—or rest generally. The joys of feasting, leisure, and worship are all richer when experienced with others. This emphasis is ancient, but more important than ever in a technological world so designed to isolate, fragment, and individualize. Shulevitz says, "If adult life is divided, the Sabbath is when we become one—with our family, with our community, with God."[7]

Note that the fourth of the ten commandments—keeping the Sabbath holy—functions like a bridge between the first three, which are about loving God, and the last six, which are about loving others. "When one enters the Sabbath," Swoboda notes, "it is as though we are loving God *and* those around us."[8]

To keep the Sabbath holy, we can't keep it to ourselves. Sabbath is not just about having quiet time between you and Jesus. We enter God's rest collectively, communing with him as we commune with his people—at church worship services, around the table, and in other expressions of resting together.

4. SABBATH IS PARTICIPATION

The centrality of communal worship on Sabbath speaks to the fact that Sabbath is not disengaged passivity but engaged participation. There is a type of Sabbath work that is not work: worshiping God, serving his church, and participating in the *shalom*-spreading activities of his kingdom.

John Walton argues that Sabbath is not a total cessation of activity but "has to do with participating in God's ordered system (rather than promoting our own activities as those that bring us order)." The work we desist from on Sabbath "is that which represents our own attempts to bring order to our lives. It is to resist our self-interest, our self-sufficiency and our sense of self-reliance."[9]

Sabbath participation communicates the reality that God's rest is not a state of frozen inaction but rather a state of security and order and peace in which we are happily under his perfect rule. God works continually, eternally upholding the cosmos by his infinite power and providence. In the Gospels, in response to accusations that his ministry and healings on the Sabbath constitute law-violating work, Jesus defends himself by identifying himself as this very same God: "In his defense Jesus said to them, 'My Father is always at his work to this very day, and I too am working'" (John 5:17). In Matthew 12 he identifies himself as "Lord of the Sabbath" (v. 8) and defends healing on the Sabbath by saying, "If any of you has a sheep and it falls into a pit on the Sabbath, will you not take hold of it and lift it out? How much more valuable is a person than a sheep! Therefore it is lawful to do good on the Sabbath" (vv. 11–12).

This doing-good work is the work of the kingdom. Its goal is the expansion of Edenic *shalom*: bringing people out of disorder and into the order of God's presence, out of spiritual exhaustion and into spiritual rest (Matt. 11:28), out of slavery and into sonship (Gal. 4:7). As we work in the service of the church on Sundays, or in acts of mercy, hospitality, and compassion done in the name of Christ and for the sake of his kingdom, we participate in the sanctified work that is at home in Sabbath rest.

5. SABBATH IS LIBERATION

One of the most powerful things Sabbath communicates is liberation. God's people are a free people: free from Pharaoh's whip, free from sin's mastery (Rom. 6:14), free from the law of sin and death (8:2). To remember the Sabbath is to remember our deliverance: "Remember that you were slaves in Egypt and that the Lord your God brought you out of there with a mighty hand and an outstretched arm. Therefore the Lord your God has commanded you to observe the Sabbath day" (Deut. 5:15).

Commenting on this passage, which shows how God ties Sabbath-keeping to freedom from slavery, Tim Keller applies the principle to contemporary life: "Anyone who cannot rest from work is a slave—to a need for success, to a materialistic culture, to exploitative employers, to parental expectations, or to all of the above. These slave masters will abuse you if you are not disciplined in the practice of Sabbath rest. Sabbath is a declaration of freedom."[10]

By practicing Sabbath, we declare our freedom from every sort of slavery that shackles us. It is deliverance from the slave driver of scarce time into the bounty of eternity. It is deliverance from stresses, enemies, and threats into the restful safety of God's peaceful presence (for example, Deut. 12:10; Josh 1:13; 2 Sam. 7:1; 1 Kings 5:4; Psalm 23). It is deliverance from restlessness into restfulness.

In *Sabbath as Resistance*, Walter Brueggemann describes the exodus as God delivering his people from "the system of endless production, in order to enter a world of covenantal fidelity," a departure from the Egyptian system of endless work "in order to dance and sing freedom." Brueggemann characterizes Sabbath as a "decisive, concrete, visible way of opting for and aligning with the God of rest." It is a sign that we have chosen God over Mammon (Matt. 6:24). Yet this choice is not easy, "for our motors are set to run at brick-making speed."[11]

In our flesh we want to keep striving, making more bricks, filling our storehouses, and hoarding our possessions to ensure a comfortable future for ourselves (Luke 12:15–20). The impulses to work hard and plan ahead are not inherently bad. But they can become all-consuming, revealing that we trust ourselves more than we trust God.

6. SABBATH IS TRUST

Trust is a prerequisite of rest. To fall asleep is to trust that you'll wake in the morning and that your world won't fall apart while you're off duty for seven hours. A baby sleeps soundly in his mother's arms because he trusts her and is at peace in this most secure spot, close to her bosom. All is well. All needs are met.

We can truly enter into Sabbath, setting aside our ambitions and anxieties for a day, only when we trust in God's goodness and provision. Trust always precedes obedience. ("Trust and Obey" is one of my favorite classic hymns!)

God emphasizes the connection between Sabbath and trust when he provides manna to the Israelites in the wilderness (Ex. 16:4–35). He gives enough for each day, and then, on the sixth day, directs the people to collect twice as much as they need because on the seventh day there will be no manna to gather. Still, some of the people go out on the Sabbath to gather manna, but they find none (v. 27). They failed to trust God. The needs of their flesh (more manna!) overtook their trust in Yahweh and obedience to his Sabbath commands.

I often struggle to practice Sabbath because I don't trust in God's provision. Even if Sunday is a day I don't work for pay, the to-dos of household work loom large: laundry, bill paying, yardwork, grocery shopping. Yet this is a posture of self-sufficiency and scarcity, believing a Sunday spent working through to-dos is more urgent than a Sunday spent reveling in

God's abundance and holiness, in community with others. What a missed opportunity.

Kelly Kapic says, without the rhythm of Sabbath rest, "we easily stick to our labor and make it our lord; we start to worship the creation rather than the Creator. . . . When we ignore our need to rest, we ignore our limits, and we end up ignoring God."[12] But if we lean in to our limits, eagerly prioritize sleep, and delight in a day of rest, we signal to a watching world that we trust a good and gracious God. He doesn't demand our constant productivity. He sustains. He provides. He is God, and we are not.

7. SABBATH IS A PREVIEW

Our weekly Sabbath is a fleeting dose of rest on earth, pointing to the unending spring of rest we will drink from in the new creation. There remains a Sabbath rest for the people of God (Heb. 4:9), and as Bavinck puts it, "Each Sabbath Day is but an example and a foretaste of it."[13]

What will this eternal Sabbath rest be like? I admit this question has perplexed me, in part because Sabbath rest in our lived experience is so inextricably tied to six days of work. We grasp the bliss of rest in this life because we know the wearying burdens of toil. So if we experience Sabbath rest eternally, how will that be enjoyable without the foil of work, something to rest *from*? Does rest have meaning apart from work?

Of course we can't know for sure what eternity will be like. I'm inclined to believe it will still include work, but a perfected form of work: a work free of thistles and thorns, burdens and toils, untarnished by sin, where our labor is not in vain (Isa. 65:23). Perhaps it will be a return to the pre-fall work God gave Adam and Eve to do. John Piper speculates that in the age to come, maybe "the line between work and play becomes almost invisible," because "work itself will be so profoundly satisfying and sweet and enjoyable that nobody will say, 'I need a weekend.'"[14]

Maybe the very concepts of work and rest will blur and merge in a beautiful way, like those stunning sunsets and daybreaks when the day and night are indistinguishable and it's such a pleasant, peaceful mixture that we wish time could stop there.

Revelation tells us we will rest from toilsome, exhausting labor in the new creation (Rev. 14:13). But it also says, "His servants will serve him" (22:3). The work we do won't be draining and obligatory but life-giving and delightful: serving the Lamb, serving others, always an outward orientation of love and building up. Work as worship.

Perhaps it will be the participation work described in point 4: the kingdom-enriching activities we do on Sabbath, the sorts of things Jesus says do not violate Sabbath prohibitions. Maybe it's the type of work so in sync with God's priorities, so peaceful under his authority, and so driven by selfless love and worship that it feels like a perpetual experience of that original seventh-day divine rest.

Blessed and holy.

Pause and Ponder

Pause

Does Sabbath as a communal activity have a place in your life? Do you fellowship weekly with believers as an act of Sabbath worship? Instead of the solitary "sabbathing" of wellness culture (rest as solo retreat or self-care), brainstorm ways you might practice

Sabbath with others: family, church family, friends, and neighbors you invite over for a Sabbath-day meal, roommates you pray and worship with once a week, and more.

Ponder

1. Based on what you've learned in this chapter, how do you feel convicted to think about or practice Sabbath differently?
2. What misconceptions about Sabbath do you see in your life or in the broader Christian culture?
3. What is the relationship between prioritizing rest and trusting God?
4. How might your Sabbath practice avoid passive disengagement but instead include active participation in God's Sabbath-appropriate, doing-good work?

12

NAPS AND SNACKS

God Is Gracious and Loving

Since God controls all that happens in his world, every meal, every pleasure, every possession, every bit of sun, every night's sleep, every moment of health and safety, everything else that sustains and enriches life is a divine gift.

—J. I. Packer, *Knowing God*

You open your hand
and satisfy the desires of every living thing.

—Psalm 145:16

Sleep, sabbath, rest, leisure. Afternoon naps, midmorning snacks. Our Creator is supremely gracious. He gives and gives and gives, shows us unmerited favor, loves us simply because he loves us. It's a grace pervasively evident in general revelation and extraordinarily manifest in special revelation: the gospel. We are saved by grace, through faith, "and this is not from yourselves, it is the gift of God—not by works, so that no one can boast" (Eph. 2:8–9).

God's grace is so mind-blowing, so amazing, that we're going to linger on it over the next three chapters, concluding this book with a worshipful reflection on the surprising ways sleep and rest point us back to the gospel itself. Chapters 13 and 14 will unpack the special mercy and grace of the gospel: the punishment we deserve but don't get (chapter 13) and the gift we get but don't deserve (chapter 14). Before we get there, though, I want to spend this chapter exploring the nature of grace: what it reveals about the kind of god God is, how common-grace gifts show up all over creation, and how it's all tied to our experience and understanding of beauty.

LEGALISM OF OPTIMIZATION AND CONTROLLABILITY

Grace stands in stark contrast to legalism: working and law-keeping to earn God's gifts. But grace also opposes subtler modes of legalism we sometimes mistake as virtues. I'm thinking of our technological age's values of optimization and controllability.

Optimization is the constant striving to improve things (including yourself); tweaking diets and dials to streamline waking life and maximize productivity; filling every spare moment with self-improvement podcasts, meditation apps, or wellness regimes to avoid dreaded downtime. A Christianized version is the (well-intentioned) notion of "redeeming the time" (Eph. 5:16 NKJV). Efficiency is the goal of optimization: eliminating excess and maximizing resources. To our modern ears, this sounds commendable, right?

The parent idea of optimization is controllability. It is the conviction that we can master the world and bend it to our will. It's modernity's driving idea: Nature can be tamed, all threats pacified. Science and technology are the engines of this quest to harness and domesticate what was once thought uncontrollable. In their extreme forms, optimization and controllability are perversions of a good thing—our God-given creative power to bring order out of chaos. And they are tendencies that go all the way back to the beginning.

Adam and Eve were given a creation mandate to fill the earth and subdue it, ruling over all creation and cultivating its resources (Gen. 1:28; 2:15). But they were also given limits (2:17). Instead of joyfully accepting their mandate within limits, they opted to transgress the boundaries, unsatisfied with a position subordinate to God's unlimited power. The fall resulted from our human ancestors' appetite for unchecked, autonomous power to optimize themselves and control the world on their own terms. And this has been a thread of fleshly temptation ever since, from Babel to Babylon to the "City of Man" spirit of optimization and controllability in contemporary life.

We see this spirit in today's technological frontiers: biohacking efforts to optimize one's body, transhumanist explorations to one day defeat mortality, fertility and abortive technologies to subject all aspects of babymaking to our convenience and control, surgical and hormonal modifications to transcend the constraints of one's biological gender, artificial intelligence to replace slow, inefficient human workers and thinkers. The list could go on.

Optimization and controllability are modern forms of legalism. Implicit in these outlooks is an understanding of what we can do in our own strength to achieve salvation. Yet this high view of our capacities leads to a burdensome, graceless life. As Hartmut Rosa puts it in *The Uncontrollability of the World*, "It is only in encountering the *uncontrollable* that we really experience the world. Only then do we feel touched, moved, alive. A world that is fully known, in which everything has been planned and mastered, would be a dead world."[1]

SLEEP AND REST: GRATUITOUS GIFTS, NOT PAYMENT OR FUEL

The optimization and controllability mindset explains everything in terms of costs and benefits: We get something good because we earn it, something bad because we deserve it. Even rest becomes subject to this logic. To justify such apparently inefficient behaviors as a solid nightly sleep or an afternoon nap, we frame these as either rewards for hard work or fuel for optimal functioning. In both cases we suck the grace out of the experience.

What if sleep, rest, and Sabbath are gifts meant to mold us to the contours of grace, rather than hacks for our wellness or rewards for our striving?

It's a natural human tendency to reframe rest in legalistic terms. In the Gospels, Jesus often challenges the Pharisaical perversion of the Sabbath into something more about dos-and-don'ts legalism than an experience of grace. "The Sabbath was made for man, not man for the Sabbath," he asserts (Mark 2:27). As Marva Dawn puts it, "To keep the Sabbath is to focus on the immensity of God's gifts to us, especially the priceless gift of salvation."[2] Walter Brueggemann compares our posture of rest to that of receiving the bread in the Lord's Supper, as a token of our salvation: "We are on the receiving end, without accomplishment, achievement, or qualification. It is a gift, and we are grateful."[3]

Rest is not a reward. Sleep is not utilitarian fuel. Rather, these are signatures of an extraordinarily generous, loving Creator who does not operate on the logic of transactional efficiency. Psalm 127:2 says God "grants sleep to those he loves." Sleep is a gift flowing out of God's abundant love, not a reward calculated from a cosmic ledger. A. J. Swoboda describes Sabbath as "a scheduled weekly reminder that we are not what we do; rather, we are who we are loved by."[4]

Sleep and rest proclaim the gospel of grace. We don't earn or deserve these gifts. God gives them. We see this truth most miraculously in our spiritual salvation (the focus of the following two chapters), but we also see it all over creation—extravagant gifts we neither earn nor deserve, but nevertheless receive: chocolate, coffee, orchids, laughter, the sound of music, the smell of a pine forest, the touch of a loved one's embrace, the way a child runs to a parent, the way a flock of birds forms, the rising of crackling campfire flames, the falling of delicate snow, the shimmering yellow of aspen leaves, the turquoise blue of a glacial lake, a baby's first cry, our every breath. Life itself.

BEAUTY'S UNCONTROLLABILITY

The thing about gifts is you can't control them. A child can send a list of hoped-for presents to Santa. But the whole point of wrapped presents on Christmas morning is the surprise: What you get is not in your control. It's often better than you can imagine.

When Adam woke up to the gift of Eve (Gen. 2:22–23)—given to him while he was in a deep sleep—he no doubt marveled at God's surprising grace. Gifts are pleasurable because we can't snap our fingers and conjure them on demand. They happen *to* us. "They fall into our laps without labor and without price," Bavinck says, commenting on God's gift of Eve for Adam. "We do not earn them nor achieve them: we get them for nothing."[5]

We can long for, pray for, and express a clear desire for a gift, as a child does with a Christmas list. But we can't control whether we get the gift. Even if you painstakingly plan a midsummer garden party or an outdoor wedding reception, there is no guarantee the weather will cooperate. You can't control the circumstances of an encounter with beauty, nor of grace.

It happens to you or doesn't; it's beyond your control. You can pray for things you want, and God desires that we do this boldly (1 John 5:14–15; Heb. 4:16) about everything (Phil. 4:6–7) all the time (1 Thess. 5:16–18).

But God's choice to give or withhold is his prerogative and a matter of grace, not merit.

Yesterday I went for a solo walk along a mountain lake. I had hoped it would be beautiful, but its beauty exceeded what I could have expected. Mid-November, yellow and orange leaves blanketed the trail, mixed with a white dusting of recently fallen snow. Fog lingered around the higher mountains flanking the lake, the lower hills decked out in burnt orange, red, and yellow. The cold beauty of a changing season was on vibrant display.

I couldn't have planned it. I won't be able to replicate it. But I received it—with breath heaving in my lungs, tears of gratitude in my eyes. I contemplated the bounty in my life, all undeserved: my wife, my children, my health, my home. Being here, right now, to witness this. All grace.

Beauty is uncontrollable. It defies our attempts at optimization and if-then transactional logic. As much as I love the beauty of a summer thunderstorm or the magic of a white Christmas, I can't control the weather. I've had incredible encounters with people, conversations over meals in which I felt deep kinship and that rare feeling of being seen and understood. But many of these encounters happened once and were never replicated in the same way with that person. Human connections are uncontrollable.

On occasion my wife and I have relished a meal at a restaurant that was so delicious we returned in subsequent years, hoping culinary lightning would strike twice. It never does. Our attempts to recreate serendipitous magic always fail. The most beautiful encounters in life—what Hartmut Rosa describes as moments of resonance—are beyond our ability to conjure or control.

We can put ourselves in the position to possibly experience resonant beauty, but we can't guarantee it. Rosa says jazz musicians experience this when they improvise together—the semicontrollability of bringing their instruments to play with a certain group of fellow artists at a certain time, but then letting uncontrollable dynamics play out. He says this is also what draws hikers to the wilderness: "Even if they know the route well, the appeal of hiking lies in the moments that cannot be controlled, in small, unexpected encounters."[6] Even if we could exert complete control, it would neuter beauty and kill the mood, argues Rosa: "Games become meaningless, music loses its appeal, love grows cold."[7]

The best artists understand this. They know their role is not to fabricate or manipulate beauty as much as to capture it as it authentically exists or unpredictably occurs, keeping the film camera rolling in the hope of capturing a resonant performance or natural phenomenon no CGI could as powerfully concoct. My favorite filmmaker, Terrence Malick, is a great example of this. His films are rife with holy moments because his creative approach is this semicontrollability mindset: being prepared with tools to capture beauty (cameras, actors, microphones) but approaching it with a posture of receptivity and gratitude for whatever unexpected beauty unfolds.

In *Only the Lover Sings*, theologian Josef Pieper says, "One of the fundamental human experiences is the realization that the truly great and uplifting things in life come about perhaps not without our own efforts but nevertheless not through those efforts. Rather, we will obtain them only if we can accept them as free gifts."[8] This is consistent with Rosa's concept of resonance, which he parallels with God's grace: Resonance "cannot be *earned*, demanded, or compelled." It rather "always has the character of a *gift*, or something that is bestowed upon or befalls us."[9]

Roger Scruton sums it up when he describes how the experience of beauty reveals "a fundamental truth about being—that being is a gift."[10] Beauty bears witness to the gift that is life and the God who is an infinitely gracious giver.

SLEEP AS SERENDIPITOUS GRACE

Sleep is an image of the uncontrollability of grace.

The best naps I've had came about unpredictably, not because I picked the right bed or couch at the right time and manufactured the perfect slumber. You can't make yourself fall asleep. When you do try to force sleep, it usually backfires. Rather, sleep happens when you give up your control, drifting away into the safety of God's provision.

I love how Pieper connects the ability to enjoy leisure with the ability to sleep. He describes a "certain serenity" in leisure that comes from our willingness to cede control. Leisure is "not the attitude of mind of those who actively intervene," he writes, "not of those who grab and grab hold, but of those who leave the reins loose and who are free and easy themselves—almost like a man falling asleep, for one can only fall asleep by 'letting oneself go.' Sleeplessness and the incapacity for leisure are really related to one another in a special sense, and a man at leisure is not unlike a man asleep."[11]

Perhaps this is one reason sleeplessness is so common in contemporary life. We struggle to give up control. We want to force sleep to fit schedules and schemata of optimization. Byung-Chul Han observes this in *Vita Contemplativa*: "The compulsion of production transforms inactivity into a form of activity in order to exploit it," such that we talk of power naps and turn even sleep and dreams into utilitarian resources that power our waking lives.

But, Han argues, far more than merely fuel for our optimization, sleep and dreams "are privileged places for truth. . . . Hands that are determined to act will not find the key to the truth. That key falls into the hands of the sleeper."[12] It's what Pieper is getting at when, commenting on Job 35:10 ("God giveth songs in the night"), he says, "God sends his good gifts and his blessings in sleep. . . . It is in these silent and receptive moments that the soul of man is sometimes visited by an awareness of what holds the world together."[13]

It boggles our modern minds to consider that our most profound encounters with truth might happen when we are inactive, even sleeping. But this is why grace itself is so scandalous. We don't want to believe our salvation is wholly out of our hands, that the greatest gift in existence can only be received, not achieved.

GRATUITOUSLY LOVING GOD

To fully embrace the beauty of sleep, leisure, and inactivity, we have to trust that God's love is more abundant than we can imagine. It doesn't abide by the logic of utility.

"God's highest value is not efficiency," Kelly Kapic writes. "It is *love*. He is more interested in beauty than speed of process; he is more concerned to lift our gaze, to provoke song, to stimulate our imaginations than he is to just get things done."[14]

This is the God of Sabbath. This is the God who created us to be in a deathlike sleeping state for a third of our lives. This is the God who created trees not only for our survival (shelter, oxygen) but for our wonder. This is the God who, as John Calvin put it, made food "to provide not only for necessity but also for our pleasure and delight."[15] We're made to taste and see God's goodness in superfluous snacks for enjoyment, not just in nutritional supplements for health; in naps for the beauty of a midday dream, not just as a battery recharge.

God's good gifts are useful, but not merely so. They're beautiful. And the ubiquitous reality of this unnecessary beauty powerfully challenges the reductionistic, optimizable, controllable tendencies of modern life, bearing witness instead to the uncapturable and manifold meaning of God and his "divine abundance in and toward the world."[16]

So take a nap. Eat a cookie. Light a campfire. Lie down to sleep. Walk on the beach. Take a friend out to lunch. Bring your camera. A notebook. A guitar. In every case, don't inflict your will like a control freak. But be ready: to snap a photo of serendipitous beauty if it comes, to scribble down a poem if inspiration strikes, to sing a new song if the mood hits, to sleep the most beautiful sleep and dream the most vivid dream.

None of it comes from you. All of it comes from God—jarring gifts of unexpected, undeserved, uncontrollable grace.

Receive it all with gratitude. Treasure it all in your heart.

Pause and Ponder

Pause

List examples of God's gracious gifts in your life: things you didn't plan, couldn't control, didn't earn but nevertheless received. Unplanned encounters. Unexpected brushes with beauty. Examples of God's generous abundant love. Write down as many as you can think of, and then add to this list in the future to keep an ongoing chronicle of the gifts God gives.

Ponder

1. Where in your life do you see the optimization or controllability mindset at work? In what sense are these postures a form of legalism?
2. What are examples of pleasures or experiences of beauty you try to engineer or manufacture? Can you think of an example (like trying to replicate an amazing meal at a restaurant) of when the folly of this became clear?
3. Why can it be hard to accept the uncontrollability of God's grace and his gifts? What practices or spiritual disciplines can help us grow in a grateful receiving posture rather than an anxious achieving posture?

13

WHILE YOU WERE SLEEPING

God Is Sovereign and Merciful

Go to sleep in peace. God is awake.
—Victor Hugo to Savinien Lapointe, March 1841

In peace I will lie down and sleep,
for you alone, LORD,
make me dwell in safety.
—Psalm 4:8

Sleep is a mercy. Nightly we enter a vulnerable, unguarded, out of our control, deathlike state and yet wake again to new life. Whatever happens in the night, there are new mercies in the morning.

Shouldn't we recognize this as miraculous?

Many of us in the modern world don't. We sleep largely in climate-controlled, secure homes where medicinal aid is just a nightstand away. Our needs are met. The dangers of sleep are held at bay, the perils of night largely out of sight and mind.

For most of human history until very recently, the perils of night were unavoidable and the scary vulnerabilities of sleep were a fact of life. Sleep didn't just mimic death in the way a sleeping body looks. Sleep was often the *occasion* of death because of an array of threats posed by poor sleeping conditions and nonexistent security.

Modern life buffers us from many of those old threats. Yet even in the affluent modern West there are circumstances when we do experience the vulnerability of sleep and don't take good sleep for granted. For sufferers of sleep-disrupting maladies, the mercy of good sleep is real. For unhoused people on the streets, or for those in such poverty that comfortable beds and safe housing aren't accessible, the mercy of good sleep is real. As we lie down to sleep in a bed with a roof over our heads, it's good to remember that more than 300 million people in the world don't have any sort of shelter.[1] For them, safe sleep can be a desperately elusive mercy.

And for parents of young children—especially newborns—the mercy of a peaceful, long stretch of uninterrupted sleep is real! I've felt this mercy. Kira and I had four kids in a seven-year span. Parents of babies know sleep is both precious and fragile. You rock the fussy infant to sleep in your arms, doing your best to delicately place them back in their crib, but inevitably the transition wakes them. The process starts over. Or you wake in the night to a child's whimper: a night terror, a wet bed, a painfully stuffy nose, a barking cough, an upset tummy (sometimes resulting in 2:00 a.m. projectile puking from the top bunk bed).

The grief of sick babies is what made the perilous nature of nighttime real to me. There is little scarier as a parent than a child with RSV or croup and the fearful prospect that their breathing might worsen at night. On those nights—and I've been there several times—you turn the monitor up and sleep fitfully, dreading what night might bring. But this fear makes the mercy of morning's sunrise especially sweet. Sometimes we've had multiple sick kids and have gone to bed expecting a long, restless night. But eight hours later we wake and marvel at what didn't transpire. Surprised by peace, we find the morning is all the more merciful. A sovereign God kept watch. He gave our family rest we didn't expect or deserve.

This is a lesson sleep teaches. Much can go wrong at night; waking up is never guaranteed. We neither control nor earn peaceful passage through the perilous night. It's a mercy granted us by a good and sovereign God.

PERILOUS NIGHT, HOPELESS PLIGHT

It was probably easier to appreciate the mercy of a safe, restorative sleep in the premodern world. This was a world without electric-light switches to flip on when something went bump in the night, a world without central heating and home security systems, a world without 911 and 24-7 emergency services.

It was a scary world at night.

In his fascinating book *At Day's Close: Night in Times Past*, historian Roger Ekirch describes how frightening nighttime was prior to the Industrial Revolution. The nightscape was "a forbidding place plagued by pestilential vapors, diabolical spirits, natural calamity, and human depravity, the four horsemen of the nocturnal apocalypse."[2] Illnesses like influenza and tuberculosis worsened at night when immune systems weakened. Sickly children (as well as adults) routinely didn't survive the night. In homes warmed by manually kept fires and stoves, waking up to house fires was common. The threat of home robbery increased after dark. Spiritual dangers of nighttime were also feared. As darkness fell, many assumed demons and other nefarious spiritual forces increased their predatory activity. Early modern slumber was thus "highly vulnerable to intermittent disruption," argues Ekirch, who cites frequent descriptors of sleep in that era as "restless," "troubled," and "frighted."[3]

Preindustrial people didn't view dusk with delight. It triggered fear. At sunset people didn't pause to poetically contemplate the beauty. They rushed home before darkness set in. Nightfall back then gave rise to the idiom "shutting-in."[4] In a world without artificial lighting, being in your home at night was scary enough, but being outside in the open darkness was terrifying and dangerous.

In this old world, when night was more tangibly fraught with peril, people knew to turn to God for protection. The common nighttime prayer "Now I lay me down to sleep, / I pray the Lord my soul to keep" dates to the Middle Ages. Faith was an important part of people's sense of security, Ekirch observes: "Seldom was God's protection more valued than at night. . . . 'By night,' affirmed the poet Edward Young, 'an atheist half-believes a God.'"[5]

Maybe waning belief in God in the twentieth century dovetailed with modern technologies (electric lighting, healthcare advances) that tamed night's frights. Why pray for the Lord's protection when technology brought the unpredictable nocturnal world more under our control?

But we delude ourselves if we think all of night's dangers have been vanquished. In 2021 ninety-eight people in Surfside, Florida, perished when their condominium collapsed around 1:22 a.m. In 2016 a strong earthquake struck central Italy at 3:36 a.m., killing more than two hundred people as they still slept in bed. Every year, thousands of babies die for unknown reasons in their sleep.[6] Thousands of children and young adults (including a high school friend of mine) die in their sleep from sudden arrhythmic death syndrome (SADS), a genetic heart defect typically undiscovered until it's too late. Hundreds perish annually of accidental carbon monoxide poisoning. Entire families have died of smoke inhalation because their homes caught on fire while they slept.

Those who die in the night never go to sleep expecting it to be their last. Even the most safety-conscious, industrialized society cannot fully protect us from nocturnal vulnerability. We can die fifty different ways in the daylight, but a hundred or more ways at night.

The perils of physical vulnerability at night point to a parallel spiritual reality. We are hopeless in our sin, dead in our trespasses, hell bound in permanent darkness. We can't protect ourselves as we sleep, nor can we raise ourselves. Only God can. "But because of his great love for us, God, who is rich in mercy, made us alive with Christ" (Eph. 2:4–5). Only by God's grace can we escape the fearsome shackles of darkness and night; only he transforms us into "children of the light and children of the day" (1 Thess. 5:5). Only God is sovereign over the realm of darkness, in both the physical and spiritual senses.

GOD IS SOVEREIGN *WHILE* WE SLEEP

Sleep is a daily reminder that God is sovereign over our salvation, both temporally and eternally. We wake physically—and spiritually—only because of God's merciful initiative. He holds the world together. Every life and death. Every step and breath. Every coming and going, waking and sleeping.

Psalm 121 comforts us with the truth that the God "who watches over you will not slumber" (v. 3), "nor sleep" (v. 4). He watches over you such that "the sun will not harm you by day, nor the moon by night" (v. 6). He "will keep you from all harm" (v. 7), keeping watch "over your coming and going both now and forevermore" (v. 8).

Our never-sleeping, ever-present God stands in stark contrast to the false gods and idols, whose comforts are nonexistent. Elijah famously mocks the prophets of Baal when their god doesn't show up on Mount Carmel: "Maybe he is sleeping and must be awakened," he taunts (1 Kings 18:27).

This reassurance that God is active, in control, keeping watch while we sleep is a truth that can actually help us sleep. As one writer puts it, "We can sleep because he doesn't."[7] This is the God who has eyes on every step we take (Prov. 5:21). This is the God "who made the Pleiades and Orion, and turns deep darkness into the morning, and darkens the day into night" (Amos 5:8 ESV).

This is not a detached, deistic God who created the world but lets it run itself. Rather it's a God who created and maintains the universe: hands on, dialed in, fully aware of all things, 24-7-365. Bavinck puts it well: "His maintenance, his sustaining power, extends to all creatures: to the lilies of the field (Matt. 6:28), the birds of the sky (Matt. 6:26), and to even the hairs of the head (Matt. 10:30). Every creature exists according to its nature—as it exists and so long as it exists—through the power of God. Even as it is *of* him, so it is *through* him (Rom. 11:36)."[8]

The same God who created the phenomenon of sleep keeps watch over all sleepers. He is sovereign over everything that happens while we sleep. So as we lie awake at night, anxious about some unfinished task or ongoing burden, we join the sleepless psalmist of Psalm 102 (v. 7) in taking comfort in the God who is "enthroned forever" (v. 12), "laid the foundations of the earth" (v. 25), and will "remain the same" (v. 27).

We rest easier because we can rest assured: God's got this. He's got everything. "If we don't believe in God, sleep can terrify us because it means that no one is looking out for us," Kelly Kapic observes. Yet for believers, sleep is a reminder "that we don't sustain the world, but that God does."[9]

Any illusions that we are omnipotent dissipate as the skies darken, our eyelids droop, and we fade away into a sleeping state of disengagement and passivity. We can get some things done while we're on. Yet the planet keeps spinning and is highly productive while we are off. As Wendell Berry once put it in a poem, "By work of ours; the field is tilled / And left to grace. That we may reap, / Great work is done while we're asleep."[10]

Charles Spurgeon once said, "God gave us sleep to remind us we aren't him."[11] John Piper compares sleep to "a broken record that comes around with the same message every day: Man is not sovereign. Man is not sovereign. Man is not sovereign."[12]

I remember being in the audience at Together for the Gospel 2010 when John MacArthur delivered a memorable sermon titled "The Theology of Sleep." Commenting on the parable of the growing seed (Mark 4:26–29), MacArthur explained how the seed's sprouting while the farmer sleeps demonstrates God's sovereignty over salvation:

> The wonder of the gospel is this: You sow the gospel and you go to sleep and it grows. We have no control over that. We don't know how that happens any more than the farmer knows how that seed, which is dead, or dormant in the ground, produces abundant life. The most erudite botanist and biologist and agriculturalist cannot explain the forces of life. The only human act, our Lord is saying, is to sow and go to sleep while the crop mysteriously grows.[13]

While we sleep, God carries on in his mission. It's a mission that graciously involves us but doesn't depend on us. We can fall asleep on the job. God never does. Psalm 127:2 is one of Scripture's most famous sleep verses. It follows verse 1, which reminds us that builders labor in vain and guards stand watch in vain unless the Lord builds the house and watches over the city. It's his sovereignty, not our capability, that matters most. The psalmist then connects this idea to sleep (v. 2):

> In vain you rise early
> and stay up late,
> toiling for food to eat—
> for he grants sleep to those he loves.

Commenting on Psalm 127, Scottish theologian John Baíllíe says, "The point the psalmist is making is that we should not carry our cares and anxieties to bed with us. Beds were made for sleeping, not for worrying." Baíllíe says those who go to bed fretful are forgetting that "when they are asleep, God is wide awake." He goes on to say,

> How blessed a thing it is, then, that we are not expected to retain the conscious control of our lives by night as well as by day, but that we are allowed to lay the reins in God's hands, entrusting ourselves to his care when we are least able to care for ourselves. . . . Sleep comes best to those who most put their trust in God. That is what the psalmist means by saying "He giveth his beloved sleep." His beloved are those who trust him.[14]

Does every person who fully trusts God have perfect sleep all the time? No. Are there people who don't trust God yet manage to have great sleep? I'm sure. But Scripture makes an important connection between our ability to rest and the orientation of our trust. Trusting in fragile things—money, health, human leaders—tends to lead to restless unease. Trusting in a rock-solid, sovereign God makes it easier to rest in peace.

GOD IS SOVEREIGN *THROUGH* OUR SLEEP

God's sovereignty is displayed not only in what he's doing in the world *while* we sleep but also in what he's doing in us *through* our sleep. Psalm 139 reminds us that he knows when we rise and lie down (vv. 2–3), he knits us together in our nine-month womb slumber (v. 13), he sovereignly determines our life's span before we are conceived (v. 16), he's with us as we sleep and when we wake (v. 18).

The Bible is full of examples of God working through our sleep. We've already mentioned the deep sleep of Adam and Abraham, in which they contributed nothing as God crafted a companion and a covenant. Sometimes God forces sleep upon people to underscore mercy amid their deep vulnerability, as in the dramatic scene when David and Abishai infiltrate Saul's camp at night. Saul and all his soldiers are sound asleep "because the Lord had put them into a deep sleep" (1 Sam. 26:12). David could easily kill them but instead spares them. The God-orchestrated deep sleep in this scene makes David's mercy all the more vivid.

On numerous occasions God communicates to people in their dreams as they sleep. He warns pagan kings like Abimelech of Gerar (Gen. 20:3, 6). He reasserts his covenant promises to Jacob (Gen. 28:12–15). He orchestrates the dreams of Pharaoh, and Joseph's interpretation of them, not only to preserve Egypt through a famine but also to catalyze Joseph's rise to power (Genesis 41).

Sometimes God works through our lack of sleep, as when he

kept Asaph awake (Ps. 77:4) or when he used the Persian king's sleeplessness (Esth. 6:1) to set things in motion that saved Mordecai and his people. I've had middle-of-the-night stretches of unwanted wakefulness when an idea or conviction came to me that God clearly put there. As annoying as these can't-sleep moments are, maybe we should pay attention to them. Perhaps God is trying to get our attention. This is not to say sleep struggles are good or that their causes aren't things we should address. But certainly sleeplessness is included in the "all things" God is capable of working for our good (Rom. 8:28).

God's sovereign work doesn't depend on our being awake or aware. This can be a frustrating part of faith. We want to know, see, understand the things God is doing in us and through us, let alone in the world. But we're only ever aware of an infinitesimal part of them. As John Piper famously tweeted, "God is always doing ten thousand things in your life, and you may be aware of three of them."[15] As the "Way Maker" bridge lyric repeats, "Even when I don't see it, you're working. . . . You never stop working."

We stop working. We sleep. God doesn't. We sow our seeds but then let the ground rest; God gives the sprout of life.

SLEEP AS AN ACT OF FAITH

In my childhood Baptist church, during the invitation time we often sang "I Surrender All." It's an appropriate hymn as people make decisions to follow Jesus. Salvation involves our surrender to a posture of trust and humble receptivity: "May thy Holy Spirit fill me / May I know thy power divine."

Sleep is a nightly image of this. It's an invitation to practice the posture of surrendered trust. As A. J. Swoboda puts it, "Sometimes to do nothing, to sleep, requires the most active trust in God."[16]

As we lie down to sleep, we give our mental anxieties and physical exhaustions to God, trusting him to tend to our burdens and restore us in the death of night, reviving us every morning. Every lying down to sleep is an enactment of the death and resurrection cycle of our salvation. We give up any notion of saving ourselves as we drift off to sleep. We can only trust that God will preserve us through the night, as he did the Israelites behind the bloodstained doors in Egypt through that terrifying night of wailing (Ex. 12:1–30). And we must trust not only that God will get us through night's death but also that he will deliver us to new life in the morning, as he did for the Israelites in their exodus out of Egypt and eventually to the promised land. "The Lord kept vigil that night to bring them out of Egypt" (Ex. 12:42), and he keeps vigil every night, the sovereign author and perfecter of our faith.

Do we sleep well and rest easy as an outgrowth of our trust in God, calmed by the internalized, embodied knowledge that God reigns and keeps watch over our every breath?

Maybe we should strive to be more like a sleeping baby at peace in a parent's arms. This was all of us once. We didn't know at the time just how much might go wrong in the night. We had no concept of the frailty of it all—our little lungs, life's litany of diseases and dangers, the precarious ecosystem of our cribs and the equally tenuous cosmos.

All we knew as sleeping babies was dependence on and trust in the parents who gave us life and who were with us through the night, every night. That's the simple knowledge we can practice as adults too, until the day we die: resting, sleeping, surrendering to the sovereignty of God and the saving grace of a loving Father. His strong arms cradle us in merciful safety. They are mighty to save. They rock us to sleep and raise us to new life.

Pause and Ponder

Pause

Meditate on Psalm 127:1–2. Memorize it. Write it on a notecard and put it on your mirror or dashboard. Let these verses regularly remind you of God's sovereignty while you sleep and through your sleep.

Ponder

1. When have you felt God's mercy in your sleep? What pain points in your sleeping life make you appreciate more deeply the mercy of a good night's sleep?
2. How does the "new morning mercy" of God waking us up each morning, "while we were dead in our sleep," parallel the spiritual reality described in Ephesians 2:1–5?
3. What bedtime rituals might you implement to center yourself on God's "never slumbers nor sleeps" sovereignty before you fall asleep?

14

RISE AND SHINE

God Raises the Dead

The seed is in the ground.
Now may we rest in hope
While darkness does its work.
—Wendell Berry, "The Seed Is in the Ground"

But Christ has indeed been raised from the dead,
the firstfruits of those who have fallen asleep.
—1 Corinthians 15:20

You can't wake yourself up. We rise to waking life without intention, effort, or conscious command ("wake up!") but rather by external forces: an alarm clock, a parent or spouse who shakes us awake, or (most naturally) by the gradual brightening of sunlight through a window. This daily rhythm is loaded with spiritual resonance, for we, too, do nothing to rouse ourselves spiritually. An external grace wakes us: the death of Christ that defeats our death, his resurrection that resurrects us.

The sun's rising wakes us physically. The Son's rising wakes us spiritually.

As sleep is an image of death, so waking is an image of resurrection. Every night of sleep and every waking up are reminders of gospel hope, recalling Christ's death and resurrection, rehearsing our own spiritual death and resurrection (if we are in Christ), and pointing to our future physical death and resurrection.

Our daily circadian rhythm bears witness to each of these death-to-life movements.

LIFE FROM DEATH

The idea of life from death is everywhere in creation. The devastating, widespread death of a forest because of fire is part of an ingenious natural cycle of ecosystem renewal: Ashes bring new nutrients to the soil, seeds germinate, and unfiltered sunlight helps grow the seedlings into trees. Every day at dinner we witness life from death when we consume nutrients from animals or plants that, in their deaths, give us life. Gardeners know that while severe pruning might look like death, it's an essential process for new life and fruitfulness. The death of dormancy in winter sets up the bountiful life of spring. Fallow fields are essential for sustainable agriculture. Examples abound.

Sleep expresses this too. As we saw in chapter 4, sleep—a sort of nightly death—regenerates and restores our lives in myriad ways. We've already observed how, in Adam's deep sleep, God brought forth life in the form of Eve, taken from Adam's side as he slept. Early church father Tertullian connected Adam's sleep to Christ's death: "For as Adam was a figure of Christ, Adam's sleep shadowed out the death of Christ, who was to sleep a mortal slumber, that from the wound inflicted on his side might, in like manner (as Eve was formed), be typified the church, the true mother of the living."[1]

Jesus' death on the cross and subsequent resurrection constitute history's ultimate life-from-death moment. As Bavinck puts it, "He was the grain of wheat which had to fall into the ground and die in order to bring forth fruit (John 12:24)."[2] What fruit it is! Because Christ died and rose again, death is defeated (1 Cor. 15:55–57) and we have hope of eternal life (1 Peter 1:3–9). Without Christ's resurrection, we'd still be hopelessly asleep in spiritual (and eventually physical) death. "But Christ has indeed been raised from the dead," Paul writes, "the firstfruits of those who have fallen asleep. For since death came through a man, the resurrection of the dead comes also through a man. For as in Adam all die, so in Christ all will be made alive" (1 Cor. 15:20–22).

Our spiritual waking up is possible because of Christ's sleep in death at the onset of Good Friday's Sabbath and the resurrection he secured for us when he stirred awake that first Easter dawn. Just as our consuming of the bread and wine of communion is an occasion to remember the life-from-death atonement Christ purchased for us, so might our daily rising from sleep be a reminder of this too. Tertullian recognized this. "When the body shakes off its slumber," he wrote in the early third century, "it asserts before your eye the resurrection of the dead by its own resumption of its natural functions."[3]

Often in the New Testament, those who die in Christ are in a state comparable to sleeping (John 11:11; 1 Cor. 11:30; 15:20; 1 Thess. 4:14). On several occasions Jesus refers to those he revives from death as being merely asleep: "She is not dead but asleep" (Luke 8:52); "Our friend Lazarus has fallen asleep; but I am going there to wake him up" (John 11:11). Jesus seems to want us to see how this physical rhythm he created bears witness to a spiritual truth he embodies: "I am the resurrection and the life. The one who believes in me will live, even though they die" (John 11:25).

We live because he died but lives. From Christ's darkest night, we get our brightest day. And there was evening, and there was morning.

LIGHT AND LIFE TO ALL HE BRINGS

Have you pondered the significance of Christ's resurrection happening in the early morning (Luke 24:1)? It's why churches hold sunrise services at dawn on Easter Sunday. Christ's resurrection is chronologically and thematically tied to the rising sun.

Many great movies have powerful sunrise scenes at their climax, coinciding with the plot's turn toward redemption, relief, or resolution. The ending of Joe Wright's 2005 *Pride and Prejudice*, for example, features a memorable romantic catharsis as Elizabeth Bennet (Keira Knightley) and Mr. Darcy (Matthew Macfadyen) meet in a field at sunrise, bathed in dawn's light as he declares his love for her. Michael Mann's 2004 thriller *Collateral* takes place almost entirely at night in LA's criminal underworld, but in the film's final shot we see night's darkness give way to dawn. And one of the unforgettable moments from Peter Jackson's *The Two Towers* happens when all hope seems lost after the bloody battle of Helm's Deep. Gandalf appears on his white horse as the blinding sun rises, along with Rohirrim reinforcements. It happens as he had promised: "Look to my coming at first light on the fifth day. At dawn, look to the east."

Examples like this proliferate in pop culture. Why? Because God built the world such that the sun is synonymous with resurrection and life. A sunrise is a universal symbol of hope.

The sun's daily rise triggers awakening in creatures of all kinds: humans, animals, plants. Our circadian rhythm—the body's natural clock—is kept in time by light exposure, priming us to sleep when it's dark and to be active when it's light. Further, the sun provides the warmth and illumination needed for creatures to live and grow by being active, productive, and able to secure food and shelter. The sun gives life in the form of energy: for photosynthesis in plants, harnessed by human technologies like solar panels, even absorbed by our skin and turned into vitamin D. Pause to consider God's creative genius: We have special vitamin D receptor cells that absorb sunlight and manufacture this vitamin, which is critical for building and maintaining healthy bones and supporting immune health. Sunlight helps us physically walk and move. Light gives life.

Charles Wesley, riffing on the prophecy in Malachi 4:2, included this verse in his iconic hymn "Hark! The Herald Angels Sing":

> Hail the heaven-born Prince of Peace!
> Hail the Sun of Righteousness!
> Light and life to all he brings,
> risen with healing in his wings.

He spelled it "Sun" on purpose. Scripture frequently associates Christ's coming with light's arrival (Isa. 9:2; John 1:1–9), bringing spiritual illumination to the fearsome dark, life to the dead world. "In the same way as the darkness which reigns in a house is dispelled by the entry of light," wrote early church father Basil the Great, "so death, which held human nature in its power, was annihilated by the coming of the Godhead. . . . Death reigned till the coming of Christ; but when the saving grace of God appeared and the sun of justice rose, death was swallowed up in this victory."[4]

The connection of Christ—and our salvation—to imagery of light and sun is all over the New Testament. Christ describes himself as the "light of the world" in John 8:12: "Whoever follows me will never walk in darkness, but will have the light of life." Paul connects the reality of spiritual regeneration with light: "God, who said, 'Let light shine out of darkness,' made his light shine in our hearts to give us the light of the knowledge of God's glory displayed in the face of Christ" (2 Cor. 4:6).

Paul also uses light imagery to describe the distinctiveness of believers: "children of the light and children of the day" who "do not belong to the night or to the darkness" (1 Thess. 5:5). In his letter to the Ephesians, Paul urges believers to "live as children of light," having once been in darkness but now having light in the Lord (Eph. 5:8). Living in the light means bearing the fruits of light (goodness, righteousness, and truth) and having nothing to do with the "fruitless deeds of darkness," Paul writes. He then connects this "living in the light" idea to waking up from sleep:

> Wake up, sleeper,
> rise from the dead,
> and Christ will shine on you.
>
> —*Ephesians 5:14*

Commenting on this passage, Bible scholar N. T. Wright says Paul is using sleep as a metaphor for death. Immoralities like lying, stealing, and sexual immorality are like being asleep because they "are forms of death": "They are ways of sleeping a deadly sleep. It's time to wake up, he says. Come alive to the real world, the world where Jesus is Lord, the world into which your baptism brings you, the world you claim to belong to when you say in the creed that Jesus is Lord and that God raised him from the dead."[5]

The association of waking up with morality is so powerful

that even secular artists and politicians adopt it to convey ethical awakening or coming into awareness about hard realities or grown-up responsibilities. I think of songs like Arcade Fire's generational anthem "Wake Up" or Rage Against the Machine's "Wake Up," which was memorably used in the end credits of 1999's *The Matrix*.

Or consider the fact that *woke* became a term to describe social justice awareness and activism. Yet in these usages, the biblical associations of being awake (soberness versus drunkenness, responsible moral living versus reckless immorality) are deployed with one key factor missing: hope.

Becoming awake via your own righteousness or moral enlightenment may seem inspiring. But it's actually a crushing burden. The goodness of being awake is good only if we're being sustained by a power beyond ourselves. That's where the sun imagery is, again, so helpful. In the Sun, we are energized by a distant force far greater than us; we don't depend on some sort of mini sun within us, powering our lives like a constantly depleting battery. God created us to rely on him, not ourselves: for our waking up, for our living in the light, for our shining as light to others (Matt. 5:14–16).

For believers, then, every dawn—every waking from sleep by the light of the sun—should be an occasion not to anxiously stew over what we must do but to remember what Christ did. His death and resurrection secured for us a new life, new future, new hope, new illumination.

As the sun rises, we can also see the world more clearly in the daylight. This bears witness to the new spiritual sight we have once we're regenerated. Everything should look different in light of Christ. C. S. Lewis puts it beautifully when he says, "I believe in Christianity as I believe that the sun has risen: not only because I see it, but because by it I see everything else."[6]

Rise and shine. Rise and see.

FORETASTES OF ETERNITY

We don't always go to bed with hope, however. Sometimes we go to bed in dread. Maybe it's a Sunday night, and we fear the Monday morning grind. Maybe it's the night before a major surgery or a daunting meeting at work. Maybe we're going to bed feeling guilty about something we've said or done. We all know that unsettled feeling of going to bed burdened or nervous for a day we don't want to face. This is part of life under the sun. Not every morning is idyllic.

The bedtime apprehension before a feared morning is perhaps an ominous picture and warning to those who don't know Christ. They will one day wake to a darkness that will never end—the melancholy dread of Mondays, times infinity.

The liminal space of sleep and dreams is a sort of in-between world that gives us glimpses of two potential eternal futures.

A restless, agonized night in which we desperately want peace but can't find it can feel like a glimpse of hell. So can our nightmares, those mysterious dark dreamscapes that occasionally feel demonic.

But the opposite is also true. A restful, deep sleep with pleasant or even beautiful dreams is a glimpse of heaven. So are those peaceful Saturday mornings when you slowly wake to the prospect of rest and leisure.

Think of your best morning ever. For me, it might be the morning of January 1, 2015, when my wife, Kira, and I woke up on New Year's Day in a hotel in Marseille, France. We rose to a new year, a bright blue sky, and the warmth of the Mediterranean sun. After breakfast we sat in lounge chairs outside, looking out over the Vieux Port and basking in the sun. I remember looking at Kira—a smile of sunbathed peace on her face, all four limbs sprawled out to fully absorb every ray she could—and feeling a joy so profound it bordered on sadness. It was one of those sublime, fleeting glimpses of eternal Sabbath. A rare glimpse of the perpetual *shalom* to come where gratitude is the default rather than discontentment and where burdens of every sort feel galaxies away.[7]

What's your best-morning memory? Just think, that memory is but the faintest foretaste of the eternal splendor to come.

Sometimes I wonder if our waking up in the new creation will be like that disorienting moment of waking up from a dream and recognizing reality in the light of day—like the transition of a monochromatic gray winter to the prismatic color of spring. Everything is clearer, more logical, and we're filled with relief that our dreams were just dreams. There is discontinuity but also continuity in that transition: We might partially remember our dreams; the person who was sleeping and the person now awake are the same person. So will it be in the new creation. We won't be waking to a totally different, jarringly unfamiliar world. We'll be waking to a jarringly *new* world, where we'll experience a "restored and perfected version of our familiar bodies and our familiar earth and our familiar relationships."[8]

Sometimes the entrance to waking reality hits us like a gut punch. We don't want it. We'd prefer to close our eyes and return to sleep. Our dream world was better. That won't be the case in heaven. It'll be so much better than the best dreams, the best joys we've had here—so much more real. "The world's delights," Richard Baxter writes in *The Saints' Everlasting Rest*, "are mere dreams and shadows."[9]

It's interesting that a commonality in those who've had near-death experiences (NDEs) is a report that they felt "more real than real life."[10] Maybe this is because our consciousness and perception in this life is, as Paul puts it, akin to a reflection in a mirror. The more real future will be like seeing face to face: "Now I know in part; then I shall know fully, even as I am fully known" (1 Cor. 13:12).

Our vision then will behold wonders and beauties far beyond what we see now, even as what we see now glimpses that future glory. When we see God face to face (Rev. 22:4), reality as we know it will explode into technicolor. Our souls' longing will be fulfilled: to dwell in the house of the Lord and gaze on his beauty (Ps. 27:4).

We can behold wonderful things now. In God's kindness we enjoy frequent foretastes: quiet morning coffee on a covered patio, campfire conversations amid the smells of mountain pine, sun-drenched mornings in Marseille. But they are merely glimpses, faint, derivative realities from the source material of heaven,[11] refracted light from the Sun's radiant glory, trickle-down streams from the gushing fountainhead of God's presence.

"The things we love are not merely the best this life has to offer," Randy Alcorn argues. "They are previews of the greater life to come."[12] N. T. Wright puts it this way: "Our present experience, with all its incompleteness, is meant to point us to the fact that we will one day wake up and arise from sleep. That, after all, is what resurrection is all about."[13]

RISEN TO WALK IN NEWNESS OF LIFE

God wants us to understand spiritual truths through physical realities. This is one of the reasons churches practice communion and baptism. They are physical rituals that signify spiritual realities.

Born and raised a Baptist, I can never keep my eyes dry when I watch someone get baptized through immersion. The imagery is vivid: A person is dunked backward into the water, totally plunged into the death of the water, as if they've fallen into a coffin six feet deep. But then they're pulled back out, mimicking their Savior's resurrection. Glistening with water, often with fists pumped into the air, the most joyous smile across their face. They have just declared their salvation in Christ through an embodied ritual. In the liturgy I grew up with, the words the pastor speaks as he dunks the person—"Buried with Christ in baptism"—are quickly followed, as he lifts the now-drenched person out of the water, by "risen to walk in newness of life."

It's a beautiful physical sign of the sweetest of spiritual truths. As we are in union with Christ, we die to our sinful bondage and are risen to freedom and purpose and life. Every Sunday this physical sign bears witness probably hundreds or thousands of times across the world.

Every night the physical sign of sleep—and waking up—bears witness too.

In sleep we are dead. But in the morning, we're risen to new life.

In baptism, escaping death is only half the story. We're risen to walk in newness of life, not just to be inert in the security of our salvation but activated to worship and serve Christ the rest of our days. Sleeping and waking bear witness to this too. We don't get up only to persist in rested stillness. We've survived the night, yes. But this grace empowers us to act: to work, to serve, to see and enjoy the beauty of God's world on full display in the light of day.

Pause and Ponder

Pause

What was your best morning ever? Think about the sights, smells, and other sensations of that moment. How was that morning a picture of eternal Sabbath?

Consider writing down a description, from your memory, of a particularly glorious morning. Describe it with as much poetry—or at least detail—as you can muster. Let the exercise stir your heart toward the glad morning to come when the sun will rise but never set.

Ponder

1. Have you ever thought about waking up from sleep as an image of resurrection? How might this daily ritual remind you of eternity and resurrection hope?
2. What should our lives look like in practice if we are to heed Paul's admonition to be "children of the light and children of the day" who "do not belong to the night or to the darkness" (1 Thess. 5:5)?
3. Contemplate the parallels and symbolic connections between the sun (our planet's primary source of light) and the Son (Jesus, our source of eternal life). Why is the motif of light so significant in salvation history?
4. What do you think it will be like to "wake up" in heaven when we die? Will the memories of our lives feel to us like half-remembered dreams, which feel surreal compared with the more tangible reality of waking life?

CONCLUSION

Join the Rest(istance)

> Rest is a weapon given to us by God.
>
> The enemy hates it because he wants us to be stressed and occupied.
>
> —Elisabeth Elliot

> Stand at the crossroads and look;
> ask for the ancient paths,
> ask where the good way is, and walk in it,
> and you will find rest for your souls.
> But you said, "We will not walk in it."
>
> —Jeremiah 6:16

Sometimes it takes time for the goodness of a gift to sink in. On Christmas morning, kids tear open presents and move on quickly from one surprise to the next. Often the gift that initially excited them most doesn't turn out to be their most beloved in the long run. And years later, when they are adults themselves, the gifts from their parents they'll remember won't be the Christmas-morning kind. Rather, they'll most appreciate the gifts of wisdom, presence, discipline, modeled holiness, prioritized churchgoing, and so forth. But as we grow up, we tend to take these things for granted. Sometimes we even find them tedious: "Dad, do we *really* have to go to church two times a day on Sunday, every week?"

It's kind of like this with the gifts of sleep and rest. Growing up, we often think bedtime is an intrusion on our fun. We fight naps. As we grow into adulthood and the optimization mindset takes hold, we relegate rest to a utilitarian category of battery recharging, embracing it only because we must.

But I hope this book has effectively argued that rest is far more than just useful. It's meaningful. It's a beautiful, mysterious key that unlocks bigger truths and connects many dots in God's design. It's a motif that shows up often both in special revelation (Scripture) and in general revelation (creation). It takes shape in a seventh-day Sabbath rhythm *and* a seven-hour nightly sleep rhythm. It's a gift that always comes hand in hand with another gift—work—and the goodness of both depends on their complementary relationship.

Looking closer at this motif—unpacking all the ways it bears witness to who God is and who he created us to be—fills me with wonder and worship. I hope it does for you too.

This close reading of a seemingly mundane reality—sleep and rest—might feel strange in a world where we're too rushed and too distracted to notice the wonder of everyday things. But if Christians are deemed strange for being people who think deeply and marvel enthusiastically about how God made the world, so be it. Sometimes it's good to be strange.

HOW SLEEP AND REST RESIST THE SPIRIT OF THE AGE

Let's recap a few of the ways embracing God's wise gift of rest—in its various forms—challenges the spirit of the age.

JOYFUL OBEDIENCE IN A WORLD OF RESTLESS REBELLION

The deepest sense of rest is spiritual. It's when our restless souls find rest in God, whose gracious provision of salvation we gladly accept. The deepest root of restlessness is sin: trusting in ourselves, going our own way. Autonomous freedom is the wandering way, and it's exhausting. We find rest for our souls, as the Lord says through Jeremiah, when we walk in "the ancient paths" and "the good way." We find peace when we submit to God's good rule, going with the smooth grain of his Word and the design of his world rather than against it (and getting splinters).

QUIET IN A WORLD OF DEAFENING NOISE

It's a louder than ever world: the constant hum of media, the pontificating talking heads, the screaming matches and streaming algorithms, the daily pressure to speak up and sound off. Silence is demeaned as violence. But usually silence isn't violence. It's a force for peacemaking. It's a mitigating "mute" that calms and quiets our souls. Silence is a key instrument in the rested soul's song. A rested soul has a quiet presence, and a quiet presence is disarming and inviting. So strive to be an invitational haven for a world exhausted by the clamor.

STILLNESS IN A WORLD OF CONSTANT MOTION

Digital life never stops. Stillness is anathema. On the "endless scroll," there's always more information to accumulate and amusements to consume. *Downtime* is becoming an antiquated term. All interstitial moments are now opportunities to maximize, for microbursts of productivity, for quick bites of tasty diversion. Sleep can feel wasteful. But a world of constant productivity and content snacking is soul deadening. We need space: to process inputs, to talk to God, to be still and know, to wonder, to wander, to daydream, to dwell, to sleep. A rested soul is comfortable with stillness. And stillness is critical to wisdom.

JOYFUL LABOR IN A WORLD AVERSE TO WORK

One of the underrated blessings of good sleep is that it makes waking and working more joyful. Both sides of this complementary relationship thrive when they are in healthy balance. We work better and harder when we also rest well. Often the best sleep comes after the hardest day of work. Yet in today's world, this complementary balance is at risk. For some it's at risk because they overprioritize work and underemphasize rest. For others it's the opposite: Work is a necessary evil, and a life of rest is the goal. But a workless world would be miserable, because rest would lose its meaning. Current dystopian assessments of AI suggest that a workless world is a possible future—eventually robots will make jobs optional for humans. This would be awful. In how we live, Christians should bear witness to the goodness of work and rest *together.* Rest goes awry when it's untethered from work. Sleep makes sense only in a world where it alternates with wakefulness.

COMMUNAL WORSHIP IN A WORLD OF LONELY CONSUMERISM

Everything in the iWorld is oriented around individuals. We're conditioned to curate our own tailored-to-me library of songs, Substacks, YouTube channels, and AI friends. It's all fit to me, on my terms, for my pleasure. It's lonely. To scroll alone, day after day, is wearying. What we crave is not to be isolated consumers but to be in a community consumed with something bigger: a transcendent God who deserves our worship and is what we need, rather than the fragile algorithmic idols that tempt us with what we want. A Sabbath-shaped life is a life of communal, bigger-than-me worship—inviting scattered consumers into a God-formed family of true rest, true connection, true contentment. Lean in to the church's potential to be a "contrast society where the world learns what true rest is."[1]

ACCEPTANCE OF LIMITS IN A WORLD OF DELUSIONAL DEFIANCE

From biohacking to transhumanism, gene editing to puberty blocking, modern technology everywhere feeds our delusional aspirations to godlike power and control. We start to believe it's possible—even advisable—to do away with all creational limits: our mortality, our gendered specificity, our need to sleep, our finite knowledge. The new frontiers of AI promise to expand this lure of limitlessness, forging a world where some believe superintelligent machines will one day cure every cancer, solve every problem, and sell some form of immortal human consciousness. Resist this ancient lie. Don't just begrudgingly accept limits such as rest and sleep. Embrace them. Follow Tish Harrison Warren's advice and relish sleep "as not only necessary but as an embodied response to the truth of Scripture: we are finite, weak creatures who are abundantly cared for by our strong and loving Creator."[2]

ABUNDANCE IN A WORLD OF SCARCITY

As much as the digital world promises "have it your way" abundance (same-day delivery, instant Spotify access to any song), the irony is most people operate out of fear and scarcity. Life's sped-up pace worsens our existential anxiety. Our overexposure to all we don't have cultivates a glass-half-empty discontent that spurs us to strive harder. We can't find peace because there's always more. If we don't get after it, we'll be left behind. It's the rat race, keeping up with the Joneses. It's the hoarding-manna mindset (Ex. 16:16–30).

But Christians should operate out of a restful abundance. We trust God's provision. We are shaped by his grace. We enjoy God's gifts (including the gift of time); we don't idolize or hoard them. We live not with bucket-list urgency but with *Sehnsucht* anticipation. We'll never taste and see every good pleasure and beauty in this life. That's okay. What little we do get to taste and see is a sacramental sign pointing to our promised future: "pleasures forevermore" (Ps. 16:11 ESV).

TRUSTING GOD IN A WORLD OF SELF-RELIANCE

Do it yourself. Follow your heart. Look within. Trust your gut. Be who you want to be. Today's empowerment slogans are meant to instill courage and hope. In reality they kill us. To be your own compass is to wander in the wilderness. Eventually you'll run out of water. But to submit to God's compass, to follow his map, will lead you to a promised land of rest and replenishment: living water that permanently quenches thirst (John 4:13–14).

'Tis so sweet to trust in Jesus. 'Tis so sweet to find refuge not in myself, but in "the rock that is higher than I" (Ps. 61:2). 'Tis so sweet to go to sleep trusting in the one who keeps watch in the night (Ps. 121:4). 'Tis so sweet to "rise before dawn and cry for help," having "put my hope in your word" (Ps. 119:147). Do not lean on your own understanding. Trust in God with all your heart. Accept his invitation into rest.

CHOOSE THIS DAY

Choose this day whom you will serve. Will it be the God of abundant grace or the idol of optimize-yourself legalism? Will it be the Prince of Peace or the algorithmic agents of anxiety? Will it be the

Creator, who crafted you to remember your death each night as you sleep, or will it be the ancient serpent, who says, "You will *not* certainly die" (Gen. 3:4)?

Our habits of rest, sleep, and Sabbath give embodied form to our choice to serve God. They are markers of our trusting submission, our gospel assurance, our awestruck worship, and they leave an impression on others.

My dad modeled this for me as I grew up. He went to bed early and woke up around 6:00 a.m. every day—and never liked when we kids were out super late. It annoyed me at the time. I thought his rigid sleep schedule was a bit weird. But his presence in the home was steady in part because he was rested. I never remember him acting exhausted or weary, though I'm sure he was at times. His deep trust in the Lord manifested in his words *and* his behavior, the very way he carried himself as a calm and peaceful—but never lazy—presence. He spent Sundays serving faithfully in church (often morning and evening services) and resting at home with his family. He and my mom set a restful tone in our home that shaped me deeply. As a parent myself now, I aspire to do the same for my own household. I want to be well rested so I can be a better blessing—a father and husband of peace, a calming presence in a hectic world, living evidence of the sweetness of trusting God.

This is the wisdom of sleep. It blesses us and it blesses others. It's a powerful spiritual sign and a timely evangelistic invitation. The unbelieving world is weary. The choice that was yours is also theirs: Come to the one who said, "I will give you rest," or keep looking for it elsewhere—to no avail. Find rest under the shade of the Son, or wilt under the scorch of the sun. Trust God or trust yourself. His will or yours.

Choose this day.

ACKNOWLEDGMENTS

Nothing in this book was consciously made with AI assistance. It's an entirely human, old-school work, created by me, but with the help of many other nonalgorithmic humans. My wife, Kira, deserves the most thanks, allowing me time on Saturdays (and a few writing retreat getaways) for deep, productive writing sessions. To Chet, Ira, and Helen: Thanks for giving up weekend time with Daddy so I could write this book!

I'd also love to thank the good people at Brot Coffee in Orange, California, where more than half of the words in this book were written. To David and Donna Toberty, thank you for letting me use your beautiful cabin to write a few chapters. And shout-out to the beautiful city of Santa Fe, New Mexico, where I wrote four chapters.

Thank you to others who helped read select chapters or provided valuable insights as I wrote: Mark Kohler, Noah Senthil, Jon Marshall, and Josh Butler.

To Erik Wolgemuth—thanks for being a trusted collaborator and advocate for my books over the last fifteen years.

To Kyle Rohane and the whole team at Zondervan Reflective—thanks for all your efforts and kindness at every stage of this book's journey.

And to all those in my life who struggle with sleep or find themselves desperate for rest—this one's for you.

NOTES

INTRODUCTION: SLEEP TALKING: THE GOSPEL IS REST

1. C. S. Lewis, *The Weight of Glory* (1941; San Francisco: HarperOne, 2001), 29–30.
2. Abraham Heschel, *The Sabbath* (New York: Farrar, Straus, and Giroux, 1951), 16.
3. Matthew Walker, *Why We Sleep: Unlocking the Power of Sleep and Dreams* (New York: Scribner, 2017), 8.
4. John Calvin, *Institutes of the Christian Religion*, book 1, chapter 5, section 1 (Peabody, MA: Hendrickson, 2008), 4.

CHAPTER 1: SLEEP'S DEEP

1. Matthew Walker, *Why We Sleep: Unlocking the Power of Sleep and Dreams* (New York: Scribner, 2017), 5.
2. Steven W. Lockley and Russell G. Foster, *Sleep: A Very Short Introduction* (Oxford: Oxford University Press, 2012), 40.
3. Chiara Cirelli and Giulio Tononi, "Is Sleep Essential?" *PLOS Biology* 6, no. 8 (August 26, 2008): https://doi.org/10.1371/journal.pbio.0060216.
4. Lockley and Foster helpfully discuss these three arguments and counterarguments in *Sleep*, 49–53. The "restoration" argument, for example, "is sharply contradicted by the fact that during REM sleep, the brain is more active than during wakefulness and many parts of the body remain very active—such as the heart" (50). The "energy conservation" argument is weakened by the fact that the energy saved by sleep is "quite modest" such that "it seems unlikely that such a high behavioral price is paid for such small returns." Plus, energy savings would be "outweighed by the increased vulnerability to predation. Animals are at their most vulnerable when asleep, and notably during REM sleep when they are effectively paralysed" (51). Arguments against the "memory and

learning" thesis include the fact that memory and learning also occur in the absence of sleep (53).

5. Cirelli and Tononi, "Is Sleep Essential?"
6. Lockley and Foster, *Sleep*, 47.
7. Sara Protasi, "The Value of Sleeping," *Journal of the American Philosophical Association* 11, no. 2 (June 2025): 249–68, https://doi.org/10.1017/apa.2024.19.
8. For a good summary of "creational theology" in the Reformed tradition, I recommend T. M. Moore's book *Consider the Lilies: A Plea for Creational Theology* (Phillipsburg, NJ: P&R Publishing, 2005).
9. Bon Iver's song "Things Behind Things Behind Things" is from his 2025 album, *Sable, Fable.*
10. Rémi Brague, *Curing Mad Truths: Medieval Wisdom for the Modern Age* (Notre Dame, IN: University of Notre Dame Press, 2019), 55.
11. R. C. Sproul, *The Holiness of God* (Carol Stream, IL: Tyndale, 1985), 227–28.
12. John Calvin, *Institutes of the Christian Religion*, book 1, chapter 5, section 1 (Peabody, MA: Hendrickson, 2008), 16.
13. Adrian Reynolds, *And So to Bed . . . : A Biblical View of Sleep* (Fearn, Scotland: Christian Focus, 2014), 10.

CHAPTER 2: NODDING OFF

1. Byung-Chul Han, *The Burnout Society* (Stanford, CA: Stanford University Press, 2015), 8–9, 11.
2. Alain Ehrenberg, *The Weariness of the Self: Diagnosing the History of Depression in the Contemporary Age* (Montreal: McGill-Queen's University Press, 2010), 232.
3. Thomas à Kempis, *The Imitation of Christ*, ed. Susan L. Rattiner, trans. Aloysius Croft and Harold Bolton (New York: Dover, 2003), 5.
4. Miguel De Cervantes Saavedra, *Don Quixote* (1605; New York: Penguin, 1990), 906.
5. I discuss this more in my article "How Manti Te'o's Fake Girlfriend Helps Explain Transgenderism," *The Gospel Coalition*, September 9, 2022, www.thegospelcoalition.org/article/manti-teo-girlfriend-transgenderism.
6. Christine Rosen, *The Extinction of Experience: Being Human in a Disembodied World* (New York: Norton, 2024), 16–17.
7. See Scott Hubbard, "The Godliness of a Good Night's Sleep," *Desiring God*, August 6, 2023, www.desiringgod.org/articles/the-godliness-of-a-good-nights-sleep.
8. C. S. Lewis, letter to Mary Willis Shelburne (November 27, 1953), in *The Collected Letters of C. S. Lewis*, vol. 3, ed. Walter Hooper (New York: HarperCollins, 2004), 378.

9. Hartmut Rosa, *The Uncontrollability of the World* (Cambridge, UK: Polity Press, 2020), vii–viii, 37.
10. Kelly M. Kapic, *You're Only Human: How Your Limits Reflect God's Design and Why That's Good News* (Grand Rapids: Brazos, 2022), 317.
11. John Piper, "A Brief Theology of Sleep," *Desiring God*, August 3, 1982, www.desiringgod.org/articles/a-brief-theology-of-sleep.

CHAPTER 3: DEAD ASLEEP

1. Shakespeare, *The Tempest*, act 4, scene 1, II.
2. Athenagoras, *The Resurrection of the Dead*, XVI, https://ccel.org/ccel/schaff/anf02/anf02.v.iii.xvi.html?queryID=37899444&resultID=154968.
3. Ira Glass, "Fear of Sleep," *This American Life*, episode 361 (August 8, 2008), www.thisamericanlife.org/361/fear-of-sleep.
4. William Bates, *The Whole Works of the Rev. W. Bates, D.D.*, ed. W. Farmer (n.d.; repr., Harrisonburg, VA: Sprinkle, 1990), 3:247, quoted in Guy Prentiss Waters, "Why Do We Fear Death?" *TableTalk*, June 17, 2024, https://tabletalkmagazine.com/posts/why-do-we-fear-death.
5. Adrian Reynolds, *And So to Bed . . . : A Biblical View of Sleep* (Fearn, Scotland: Christian Focus, 2014), 59.
6. Megan Starr and Noah Senthil, "The Coddling of the American Funeral," *The Gospel Coalition*, November 25, 2024, www.thegospelcoalition.org/article/coddling-american-funeral.
7. Yuval Noah Harari, "Will Coronavirus Change Our Attitudes to Death? Quite the Opposite," *The Guardian*, April 20, 2020, www.theguardian.com/books/2020/apr/20/yuval-noah-harari-will-coronavirus-change-our-attitudes-to-death-quite-the-opposite.
8. Quotes in this section are from Martin Hägglund, *This Life: Secular Faith and Spiritual Freedom* (New York: Anchor, 2019), 5, 9, 13.
9. An interesting pop culture articulation of this secular faith is in season 3 of HBO's *The White Lotus*, when Carrie Coon's character delivers an existential monologue about her ongoing search for meaning: "I don't need religion or God to give my life meaning. Because *time* gives it meaning."
10. Cameron Cole, *Heavenward: How Eternity Can Change Your Life on Earth* (Wheaton: Crossway, 2024), 3.
11. Whitney K. Pipkin, *We Shall All Be Changed: How Facing Death with Loved Ones Transforms Us* (Chicago: Moody, 2024), 17.
12. Tish Harrison Warren, *Prayer in the Night: For Those Who Work or Watch or Weep* (Downers Grove, IL: InterVarsity Press, 2021), 122.
13. Bobby Jamieson, *Everything Is Never Enough: Ecclesiastes' Surprising Path to Resilient Happiness* (Colorado Springs: WaterBrook, 2025), 103.

CHAPTER 4: BEST MEDICINE

1. Margaret Thatcher, who famously slept only five hours a night, is often credited with saying, "Sleep is for wimps."
2. Tertullian, *A Treatise on the Soul*, XLIII, https://catholiclibrary.org/library/view?docId=/Synchronized-EN/anf.000065.Tertullian.ATreatiseontheSoul.html;chunk.id=00000089.
3. Steven W. Lockley and Russell G. Foster, *Sleep: A Very Short Introduction* (Oxford: Oxford University Press, 2012), 1.
4. Matthew Walker, *Why We Sleep: Unlocking the Power of Sleep and Dreams* (New York: Scribner, 2017), 108.
5. William Shakespeare, *Macbeth*, act 2, scene 2.
6. "Getting Good Sleep Could Add Years to Your Life," American College of Cardiology, press release, February 23, 2023, www.acc.org/About-ACC/Press-Releases/2023/02/22/21/35/Getting-Good-Sleep-Could-Add-Years-to-Your-Life.
7. Andrea Rice, "Sleeping In on Weekends May Lower Your Heart Disease Risk by 20%," *Healthline*, August 29, 2024, www.healthline.com/health-news/weekend-sleep-lower-heart-disease-risk.
8. Walker, *Why We Sleep*, 7.
9. Antonio Zadra and Robert Stickgold, *When Brains Dream: Exploring the Science and Mystery of Sleep* (New York: Norton, 2021), 60.
10. Mark Kohler, Zoom interview with the author, recorded on November 18, 2024.
11. Zadra and Stickgold, *When Brains Dream*, 63.
12. Lockley and Foster, *Sleep*, 52–53.
13. Zadra and Stickgold, *When Brains Dream*, 72.
14. Walker, *Why We Sleep*, 132.
15. Walker, *Why We Sleep*, 227.
16. Walker, *Why We Sleep*, 207.
17. Walker, *Why We Sleep*, 7, 210.
18. John Baíllíe, "The Theology of Sleep," in *Christian Devotion: Addresses by John Baíllie* (London: Oxford University Press, 1962), https://pmoser.sites.luc.edu/johnbailliearchive/BaillieChristianDevotion.html#sleep.
19. Walker, *Why We Sleep*, 39.
20. Lockley and Foster, *Sleep*, 133.
21. Short sleep is associated with more than a 45 percent greater risk of fatal and nonfatal coronary heart disease (Walker, *Why We Sleep*, 165).
22. Lockley and Foster observe, "It is interesting to note that since the 1960s, reported sleep duration has decreased while the rate of obesity has simultaneously increased" (Lockley and Foster, *Sleep*, 93).

23. "Men who report sleeping too little—or having poor quality sleep—have a 29 percent lower sperm count than those obtaining a full and restful night of sleep" (Walker, *Why We Sleep*, 179).
24. Walker, *Why We Sleep*, 296.
25. Baíllíe, "Theology of Sleep."
26. Wendell Berry, "A man with some authentic worries," 1995, I, *This Day: Collected and New Sabbath Poems 1979–2012* (Berkeley, CA: Counterpoint, 2013), 157.

CHAPTER 5: PERCHANCE TO DREAM

1. George MacDonald, "The Imagination: Its Function and Its Culture" (1867), George MacDonald Society, https://george-macdonald.com/essays_sermons/the_imagination.html.
2. Antonio Zadra and Robert Stickgold, *When Brains Dream: Exploring the Science and Mystery of Sleep* (New York: Norton, 2021), 51.
3. Zadra and Stickgold, *When Brains Dream*, 43.
4. Steven W. Lockley and Russell G. Foster, *Sleep: A Very Short Introduction* (Oxford: Oxford University Press, 2012), 9.
5. J. Allan Hobson, *Dreaming: An Introduction to the Science of Sleep* (Oxford: Oxford University Press, 2002), 6.
6. Zadra and Stickgold, *When Brains Dream*, 160.
7. Zadra and Stickgold, *When Brains Dream*, 91.
8. Zadra and Stickgold, *When Brains Dream*, 171–72.
9. Hobson, *Dreaming*, 86.
10. Zadra and Stickgold, *When Brains Dream*, 80.
11. Zadra and Stickgold, *When Brains Dream*, 270.
12. Deirdre Barrett, "Dreams and Creative Problem-Solving," *Annals of the New York Academy of Sciences* 1406, no. 1 (October 2017): 66, https://doi.org/10.1111/nyas.13412.
13. Walker, *Why We Sleep*, 220.
14. This is one reason why Christians should be wary of the "instant answers" and "instant creation" capabilities AI offers. If God values process in creation and we image God, we should value process too. Even if it's possible to give a prompt to AI and get a masterful result that would have taken us weeks or years, we ought to consider what's lost when slow, deliberate, creative processing is bypassed or rendered unnecessary by efficient technologies.
15. Zadra and Stickgold, *When Brains Dream*, 115.
16. Zadra and Stickgold, *When Brains Dream*, 111.

17. Zadra and Stickgold, *When Brains Dream*, 265.

CHAPTER 6: ONLY A DREAM?

1. John Newton, *Memoirs of the Rev. John Newton* (London: L. B. Seeley, 1820), 19.
2. Darren Carlson, "When Muslims Dream of Jesus," *The Gospel Coalition*, May 31, 2018, www.thegospelcoalition.org/article/muslims-dream-jesus.
3. Mark Kohler, Zoom interview with the author, recorded on November 18, 2024.
4. *The Nightmare*, directed by Rodney Ascher (FilmRise, 2015).
5. Tertullian, *A Treatise on the Soul*, XLVII, https://catholiclibrary.org/library/view?docId=/Synchronized-EN/anf.000065.Tertullian.ATreatiseontheSoul.html;query=heathen;chunk.id=00000097.
6. Gregory of Nyssa, *Dogmatic Treatises*, XIII, "A Rationale of Sleep, of Yawning, and of Dreams," in *Nicene and Post-Nicene Fathers*, https://ccel.org/ccel/schaff/npnf205/npnf205.x.ii.ii.xiv.html.
7. Augustine, *Confessions*, book 10, chapter 30.
8. John Piper, "How Do I Respond to Sexual Dreams?" *Ask Pastor John*, episode 1417 (January 6, 2020), www.desiringgod.org/interviews/how-do-i-respond-to-sexual-dreams.
9. For a fascinating philosophical reflection on lucid dreaming (and other dreaming curiosities), I recommend Richard Linklater's 2001 animated film, *Waking Life*.
10. Antonio Zadra and Robert Stickgold describe lab studies that involve lucid dreamers communicating with researchers during periods of lucidity while in REM sleep "by using predetermined eye-movement signals" that allow them to "time-stamp" when they start and finish tasks in their dreams. These studies have provided "incontrovertible evidence of lucid dreaming" (Antonio Zadra and Robert Stickgold, *When Brains Dream: Exploring the Science and Mystery of Sleep* [New York: Norton, 2021], 231).
11. Stephanie Kulke and Kristin Samuelson, "Leveraging the Power of Lucid Dreams," *Northwestern Now*, October 31, 2024, https://news.northwestern.edu/stories/2024/10/leveraging-the-power-of-lucid-dreams.
12. Richard Baxter, "Directions Against Sinful Dreams," *Practical Works*, vol. 3 (London: James Duncan, 1830), 470.
13. John Baíllíe, "The Theology of Sleep," in *Christian Devotion: Addresses by John Baíllíe* (London: Oxford University Press, 1962), https://pmoser.sites.luc.edu/johnbailliearchive/BaillieChristianDevotion.html#sleep.

14. Zadra and Stickgold, *When Brains Dream*, 122, 127.

CHAPTER 7: SLEEPING THROUGH STORMS

1. Benjamin L. Gladd, "Sleep Like a King: Why Jesus Slept Before Calming the Storm," *The Gospel Coalition*, August 16, 2024, www.thegospelcoalition.org/article/jesus-slept-calming-storm.
2. For more on this topic, I recommend Mark Sayers' *A Non-Anxious Presence: How a Changing and Complex World Will Create a Remnant of Renewed Christian Leaders* (Chicago: Moody, 2022).
3. Seth Troutt, "Rightly Ordered . . . Anxiety?" *The Gospel Coalition*, October 20, 2024, www.thegospelcoalition.org/article/rightly-ordered-anxiety.
4. Adrian Reynolds, *And So to Bed . . . : A Biblical View of Sleep* (Fearn, Scotland: Christian Focus, 2014), 81.
5. Jeremiah Burroughs, *The Rare Jewel of Christian Contentment* (1648; Banner of Truth Trust, 1979).
6. Alain Ehrenberg, *The Weariness of the Self: Diagnosing the History of Depression in the Contemporary Age* (Montreal: McGill-Queen's University Press, 2010), 218–19.
7. Justin Taylor, "An Analysis of One of the Greatest Sentences Ever Written," *The Gospel Coalition*, March 9, 2017, www.thegospelcoalition.org/blogs/justin-taylor/an-analysis-of-one-of-the-greatest-sentences-ever-written.

CHAPTER 8: HAMMOCKS AND HUMMINGBIRDS

1. Quoted in Ben Palpant, *An Axe for the Frozen Sea: Conversations with Poets About What Matters Most* (Nashville: Rabbit Room Press, 2024), 113, 119.
2. D. A. Carson, *Scandalous: The Cross and Resurrection of Jesus* (Wheaton: Crossway, 2010), 147.
3. Walter Brueggemann, *Sabbath as Resistance: Saying No to the Culture of Now* (Louisville, KY: Westminster John Knox, 2014), 45, 81.
4. Brueggemann, *Sabbath as Resistance*, 85.
5. Kelly M. Kapic, *You're Only Human: How Your Limits Reflect God's Design and Why That's Good News* (Grand Rapids: Brazos, 2022), 129.
6. Brueggemann, *Sabbath as Resistance*, 67.
7. Byung-Chul Han, *The Scent of Time: A Philosophical Essay on the Art of Lingering*, trans. Daniel Steuer (Cambridge, UK: Polity Press, 2017), 87.
8. Martin Schleske, *The Sound of Life's Unspeakable Beauty*, trans. Janet Gesme (Grand Rapids: Eerdmans, 2020), 28.

9. Richard Baxter, *The Saints' Everlasting Rest*, updated and abridged by Tim Cooper (Wheaton: Crossway, 2022), 153.
10. Byung-Chul Han, *Vita Contemplativa: In Praise of Inactivity*, trans. Daniel Steuer (Cambridge, UK: Polity Press, 2024), 55.
11. John Calvin, *Institutes of the Christian Religion*, book 1, chapter 5, section 1 (Peabody, MA: Hendrickson, 2008), 16.
12. Amy Baik Lee, *This Homeward Ache: How Our Yearning for the Life to Come Spurs On Our Life Today* (Brentwood, TN: B&H, 2023), 178.
13. Schleske, *Unspeakable Beauty*, 29.

CHAPTER 9: ON THE SEVENTH DAY

1. Guy Prentiss Waters, *The Sabbath Rest and Hope for the People of God*, Short Studies in Biblical Theology (Wheaton: Crossway, 2022), 28.
2. R. C. Sproul, *The Holiness of God* (Carol Stream, IL: Tyndale, 1985), 261.
3. Waters, *Sabbath Rest*, 31.
4. Abraham Heschel, *The Sabbath* (New York: Farrar, Straus, and Giroux, 1951), 9.
5. Heschel, *Sabbath*, 16.
6. Tim Keller, "Wisdom and Sabbath Rest," *Redeemer City to City*, July 13, 2021, https://redeemercitytocity.com/articles-stories/wisdom-and-sabbath-rest.
7. Judith Shulevitz, *The Sabbath World: Glimpses of a Different Order of Time* (New York: Random House, 2010), 217.
8. John H. Walton, *The Lost World of Adam and Eve: Genesis 2–3 and the Human Origins Debate* (Downers Grove, IL: IVP Academic, 2015), 47.
9. John H. Walton, Victor H. Matthews, and Mark W. Chavalas, *The IVP Bible Background Commentary: Old Testament* (Downers Grove, IL: InterVarsity Press, 2000), 30.
10. John H. Walton, *The Lost World of Genesis One: Ancient Cosmology and the Origins Debate* (Downers Grove, IL: IVP Academic, 2009), 74.
11. Walton, *Lost World of Adam and Eve*, 48.
12. Walton, Matthews, and Chavalas, *IVP Bible Background Commentary: Old Testament*, 30.
13. John Sailhamer, *Genesis Unbound: A Provocative New Look at the Creation Account* (Colorado Springs: Book Villages, 1996), 157.

CHAPTER 10: CREATION WORKS AND SLUMBERS

1. Matthew Walker, *Why We Sleep: Unlocking the Power of Sleep and Dreams* (New York: Scribner, 2017), 63–64.

2. David Flusfeder, "Perchance to Dream," *Prospect*, February 29, 2008, www.prospectmagazine.co.uk/opinions/52204/perchance-to-dream.
3. For more on this, see my article "'Severance' and Pop Culture Visions of Hell," *The Gospel Coalition*, February 21, 2025, www.thegospelcoalition.org/article/severance.
4. Aristotle, *On Sleep and Sleeplessness* (350 BCE), trans. J. I. Beare, https://classics.mit.edu/Aristotle/sleep.html.
5. Walker, *Why We Sleep*, 56.
6. Abraham Heschel, *The Sabbath* (New York: Farrar, Straus, and Giroux, 1951), 14.
7. Byung-Chul Han, *Vita Contemplativa: In Praise of Inactivity*, trans. Daniel Steuer (Cambridge, UK: Polity Press, 2024), 2–3.
8. Josef Pieper, *Leisure: The Basis of Culture*, trans. Alexander Dru (1952; San Franciso: Ignatius, 2009), 50.
9. Tish Harrison Warren, *Liturgy of the Ordinary: Sacred Practices in Everyday Life* (Downers Grove, IL: IVP, 2016), 150–51.
10. Eugene H. Peterson, *Working the Angles: The Shape of Pastoral Integrity* (Grand Rapids: Eerdmans, 1987), 68.
11. Gregory of Nyssa, *Dogmatic Treatises*, XIII, "A Rationale of Sleep, of Yawning, and of Dreams," in *Nicene and Post-Nicene Fathers*, https://ccel.org/ccel/schaff/npnf205/npnf205.x.ii.ii.xiv.html.
12. Fred Sanders, *The Deep Things of God: How the Trinity Changes Everything* (Wheaton: Crossway, 2010), 96.
13. D. A. Carson, *The Difficult Doctrine of the Love of God* (Wheaton: Crossway, 2000), 39.
14. Carson, *Difficult Doctrine*, 40.

CHAPTER 11: REMEMBER THE SABBATH

1. Herman Bavinck, *The Wonderful Works of God* (Glenside, PA: Westminster Seminary Press, 2019), 198.
2. Judith Shulevitz, *The Sabbath World: Glimpses of a Different Order of Time* (New York: Random House, 2010), 63.
3. Abraham Heschel, *The Sabbath* (New York: Farrar, Straus, and Giroux, 1951), 29.
4. A. J. Swoboda, *Subversive Sabbath: The Surprising Power of Rest in a Nonstop World* (Grand Rapids: Brazos, 2018), 100.
5. Eugene H. Peterson, *As Kingfishers Catch Fire: A Conversation on the Ways of God Formed by the Words of God* (Colorado Springs: WaterBook, 2017), 14.
6. Heschel, *Sabbath*, 54.
7. Shulevitz, *Sabbath World*, 6.

8. Swoboda, *Subversive Sabbath*, 110.
9. John H. Walton, *The Lost World of Adam and Eve: Genesis 2–3 and the Human Origins Debate* (Downers Grove, IL: IVP Academic, 2015), 48.
10. Tim Keller, "Wisdom and Sabbath Rest," *Redeemer City to City*, July 13, 2021, https://redeemercitytocity.com/articles-stories/wisdom-and-sabbath-rest.
11. Walter Brueggemann, *Sabbath as Resistance: Saying No to the Culture of Now* (Louisville, KY: Westminster John Knox, 2014), 18, 10, 19.
12. Kelly M. Kapic, *You're Only Human: How Your Limits Reflect God's Design and Why That's Good News* (Grand Rapids: Brazos, 2022), 220.
13. Bavinck, *Wonderful Works of God*, 198.
14. John Piper, "Will We Work in Eternity?" *Ask Pastor John*, episode 1973, September 4, 2023, www.desiringgod.org/interviews/will-we-work-in-eternity.

CHAPTER 12: NAPS AND SNACKS

1. Hartmut Rosa, *The Uncontrollability of the World* (Cambridge, UK: Polity Press, 2020), 2.
2. Marva J. Dawn, *Keeping the Sabbath Wholly: Ceasing, Resting, Embracing, Feasting* (Grand Rapids: Eerdmans, 1989), 130.
3. Walter Brueggemann, *Sabbath as Resistance: Saying No to the Culture of Now* (Louisville, KY: Westminster John Knox, 2014), xvii.
4. A. J. Swoboda, *Subversive Sabbath: The Surprising Power of Rest in a Nonstop World* (Grand Rapids: Brazos, 2018), 17.
5. Herman Bavinck, *The Wonderful Works of God* (Glenside, PA: Westminster Seminary Press, 2019), 171.
6. Rosa, *Uncontrollability*, 55–56.
7. Rosa, *Uncontrollability*, 106.
8. Josef Pieper, *Only the Lover Sings: Art and Contemplation*, trans. Lothar Krauth (San Francisco: Ignatius, 1990), 25.
9. Rosa, *Uncontrollability*, 59.
10. Roger Scruton, *The Soul of the World* (Princeton, NJ: Princeton University Press, 2014), 139.
11. Josef Pieper, *Leisure: The Basis of Culture*, trans. Alexander Dru (1952; San Franciso: Ignatius, 2009), 47.
12. Byung-Chul Han, *Vita Contemplativa: In Praise of Inactivity*, trans. Daniel Steuer (Cambridge, UK: Polity Press, 2024), 8, 9.
13. Pieper, *Leisure*, 48.
14. Kelly M. Kapic, *You're Only Human: How Your Limits Reflect God's Design and Why That's Good News* (Grand Rapids: Brazos, 2022), 148.

15. John Calvin, *On the Christian Life: A New Translation*, trans. Raymond Blacketer (Wheaton: Crossway, 2024), 59.
16. Jeremy S. Begbie, *Abundantly More: The Theological Promise of the Arts in a Reductionist World* (Grand Rapids: Baker Academic, 2023), 216.

CHAPTER 13: WHILE YOU WERE SLEEPING

1. Daniil Filipenco, "Homelessness Statistics in the World: Causes and Facts," *DevelopmentAid*, March 27, 2025, www.developmentaid.org/news-stream/post/157797/homelessness-statistics-in-the-world.
2. A. Roger Ekirch, *At Day's Close: Night in Times Past* (New York: Norton, 2005), 56.
3. Ekirch, *At Day's Close*, 288.
4. Ekirch, *At Day's Close*, 91.
5. Ekirch, *At Day's Close*, 97.
6. According to the CDC, in 2022 there were about 3,700 sudden unexpected infant deaths (SUID) in the United States. "Data and Statistics for SUID and SIDS," Centers for Disease Control, September 17, 2024, www.cdc.gov/sudden-infant-death/data-research/data/index.html.
7. Adrian Reynolds, *And So to Bed . . . : A Biblical View of Sleep* (Fearn, Scotland: Christian Focus, 2014), 47.
8. Herman Bavinck, *The Wonderful Works of God* (Glenside, PA: Westminster Seminary Press, 2019), 160–61.
9. Kelly M. Kapic, *You're Only Human: How Your Limits Reflect God's Design and Why That's Good News* (Grand Rapids: Brazos, 2022), 215.
10. Wendell Berry, "Whatever is foreseen in joy," 1979, X, *This Day: Collected and New Sabbath Poems* (Berkeley: Counterpoint, 2013), 20.
11. Quoted in Matt Hodges, "The Merciful Theology of Sleep," *Acts29*, August 2, 2022, www.acts29.com/the-merciful-theology-of-sleep.
12. John Piper, "A Brief Theology of Sleep," *Desiring God*, August 3, 1982, www.desiringgod.org/articles/a-brief-theology-of-sleep.
13. John MacArthur, "The Theology of Sleep," sermon delivered at Together for the Gospel (April 14, 2010). Transcript at *Grace to You*: www.gty.org/library/sermons-library/GTY128/the-theology-of-sleep. Also available on YouTube: www.youtube.com/watch?v=VmwWxZQb0Yw.
14. John Baíllíe, "The Theology of Sleep," in *Christian Devotion: Addresses by John Baíllíe* (London: Oxford University Press, 1962), https://pmoser.sites.luc.edu/johnbailliearchive/BaillieChristianDevotion.html#sleep.
15. John Piper, "God Is Always Doing 10,000 Things in Your Life," *Desiring God*, January 1, 2013, www.desiringgod.org/articles/god-is-always-doing-10000-things-in-your-life.

16. A. J. Swoboda, *Subversive Sabbath: The Surprising Power of Rest in a Nonstop World* (Grand Rapids: Brazos, 2018), 180.

CHAPTER 14: RISE AND SHINE

1. Tertullian, *A Treatise on the Soul*, XLIII, https://catholiclibrary.org/library/view?docId=/Synchronized-EN/anf.000065.Tertullian.ATreatiseontheSoul.html;chunk.id=00000089.
2. Herman Bavinck, *The Wonderful Works of God* (Glenside, PA: Westminster Seminary Press, 2019), 329.
3. Tertullian, *Treatise on the Soul*.
4. Basil the Great, quoted in *Celebrating the Seasons: Daily Spiritual Readings for the Christian Year*, compiled and introduced by Robert Atwell (Harrisburg, PA: Morehouse, 2001), 54.
5. N. T. Wright, *Surprised by Hope: Rethinking Heaven, the Resurrection, and the Mission of the Church* (New York: HarperOne, 2008), 252.
6. C. S. Lewis, "Is Theology Poetry?" in *The Weight of Glory* (1941; San Francisco: HarperOne, 2001), 140.
7. Some of this paragraph is taken from my blog post "Morning in Marseille," BrettMcCracken.com, December 30, 2020, www.brettmccracken.com/blog/2020/12/20/morning-in-marseille.
8. Randy Alcorn, *Heaven* (Carol Stream, IL: Tyndale, 2004), 154.
9. Richard Baxter, *The Saints' Everlasting Rest*, updated and abridged by Tim Cooper (Wheaton: Crossway, 2022), 90.
10. Gideon Lichfeld, "The Science of Near-Death Experiences," *The Atlantic*, April 2015, www.theatlantic.com/magazine/archive/2015/04/the-science-of-near-death-experiences/386231.
11. Randy Alcorn helpfully engages Hebrews (8:5; 9:11, 24; 12:22) to argue that earth is a derivative realm and heaven is the source: "We should stop thinking of heaven and earth as opposites and instead view them as overlapping circles that share certain commonalities. . . . [Hebrews suggests that] God created earth in the image of heaven, just as he created mankind in his image. . . . Isn't it more likely that earthly realities, including cities, are derived from heavenly counterparts?" (Alcorn, *Heaven*, 53–54).
12. Alcorn, *Heaven*, 161.
13. Wright, *Surprised by Hope*, 287.

CONCLUSION: JOIN THE REST(ISTANCE)

1. A. J. Swoboda, *Subversive Sabbath: The Surprising Power of Rest in a Nonstop World* (Grand Rapids: Brazos, 2018), 165.
2. Tish Harrison Warren, *Liturgy of the Ordinary: Sacred Practices in Everyday Life* (Downers Grove, IL: IVP, 2016), 152.

Songs for Sleep

Scan the QR code to access a free Spotify playlist, curated by Brett McCracken exclusively for readers of this book.

Enjoy the playlist as a musical supplement to your reading of *The Wisdom of Sleep* or as a soothing soundtrack on draining days.